S6923

14.99.

D0274659

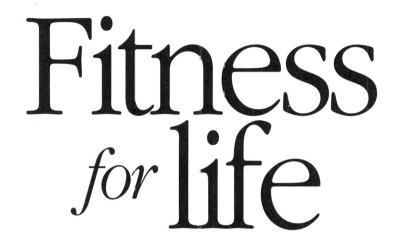

Fitness *for* life

Fitness *for* life

Susie Dinan and Dr Craig Sharp

From the Central YMCA

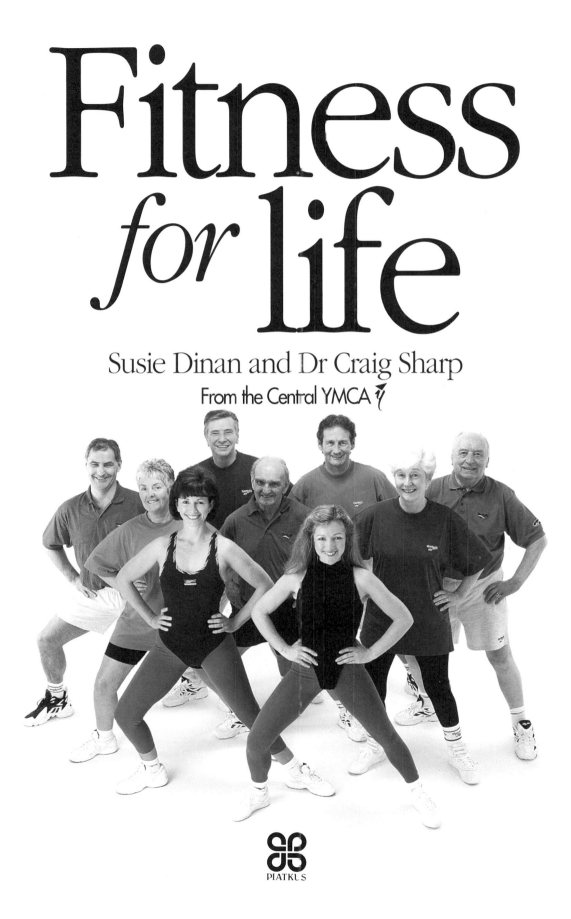

PIATKUS

First published in 1996 by
Judy Piatkus (Publishers) Ltd
5 Windmill Street, London W1P 1HF

The moral right of the authors has been asserted
*A catalogue record for this book is available
from the British Library*

ISBN 0-7499-1670-2 (hb)
ISBN 0-7499-1577-3 (pbk)

Designed by Jerry Goldie
Photographs by Jon Stewart
Image retouching by Alan Steadman

Typeset by Create Publishing Services Limited, Bath
Printed in Great Britain by Butler & Tanner Ltd, Frome and London

Contents

Acknowledgements

We would like to thank

The Central YMCA Training and Development Team.

Susie would further like to thank Jill Gaskell, Rozalind Gruben, Helen Keighley, Lesley Mowbray and Fiona Taylor Winter from Central YMCA, and colleagues at the Royal Free Hospital Medical School Department of Geriatric Medicine and the Wandsworth Community Team for People with Learning Disabilities.

She would especially like to thank Lucy Jackson, Fiona Hayes and Barbara Dale for their encouragement and support.

Thanks to Julia Lupton and Susan Boreland for their dedicated typing of the manuscript and Piatkus for their guidance and enthusiasm.

To all my extraordinary seniors at Central YMCA and The Royal Free Hospital Recreation Club for their continuing inspiration and friendship.

To my grandmother and mother, Agnes Brown and Rosemary Dinan, for their love.

Craig wishes to express his great appreciation for the inspirational example of two astonishing Scottish non-ageniarians, Ena Scott of Carluke and Naomi Mitchison of Kintyre.

Foreword

The considerable health benefits of exercise are even greater as we get older. As a result, 'More people, more active, more often' is one of the most important public health goals in the developed world. For the individual, exercise has the added attraction that it is something we can do for ourselves in order to improve our health and wellbeing. First, however, most of us require some help and guidance before we can take full responsibility for this aspect of our health.

How can the individual member of the public learn how to exercise **safely**, **effectively** and **enjoyably**? Who can tackle the very difficult, but crucial, task of bringing together the factual knowledge of medical science and the empirical knowledge of exercise practitioners and sports coaches? Who can tackle the even harder task of making this information accessible for the general reader? Enter Craig Sharp and Susie Dinan, each highly respected in their profession, and each renowned for their teaching skills. You are in safe hands!

Enjoy *Fitness For Life* and welcome to the world of better health.

Professor Archie Young
University Department of Geriatric Medicine,
Royal Free Hospital School of Medicine,
London

Central YMCA Fitness and Exercise

Central YMCA (formerly London Central YMCA) is an international organisation whose purpose is the development of mind, body and spirit for individuals of all ages and backgrounds. It has been at the forefront of keeping people fit and healthy for the past 150 years and continues today, more strongly than ever.

This philosophy, combined with a clearly identified need for well-trained exercise and fitness coaches, teachers and instructors in the community, led to the founding of Central YMCA Training and Development Operation – the UK's premier health and fitness teacher training organisation. Operating nationwide, we offer people the chance to achieve nationally recognised qualifications in more than 12 different exercise and fitness disciplines.

With core courses well established, Central YMCA Training and Development Department has expanded its training focus to encompass specialist areas of the population. One important area of development has been for the older person, a subject dealt with clearly and comprehensively in this book.

With the older adult population becoming a dominant sector in the community, there is an increasing necessity to address the exercise needs of this important group. Simply, if people are now living longer and retiring from full-time work earlier, they should have all the opportunity possible to enable them to enjoy this extended life to the full. The public in general are now positively encouraged to be more active, more often.

The focus of our development has been to increase the provision and standard of provision of exercise for this age group. To meet this need, Central YMCA worked with gerontologists, geriatricians and specialist physiotherapists to develop its nationally recognised training programme for exercise in this field. To date there are over 550 YMCA specialist teachers who run exercise classes for this age group in leisure centres, health clubs, YMCAs, halls and community centres all over the country.

The promotion of activity for life will ensure a better quality of life for the older person.

Introduction

This book is a celebration of active living and its positive effects on our bodies, our health and enjoyment of life. It is, in fact, a celebration not of actual age but of 'Body Age', which is what really counts. Each of us has a body that is unique and no two bodies age at the same rate. Only one thing is sure – we need to keep moving, for all living tissues benefit from exercise and shrink, weaken and break down when movement stops. This is the case whether you are in your twenties, forties, sixties or eighties.

Growing older is a natural and inevitable process, becoming disabled through inactivity is not.

Inactivity and ageing

Space travel has revealed that after only a few days in a weightless environment – the ultimate in inactivity – astronauts, some of the fittest humans in the universe, showed significant signs of what we have traditionally associated with ageing. They had high blood pressure, deconditioned muscles, more fragile bones; they experienced breathlessness and balance problems – all of which returned to normal after a period of activity training. Imagine then the effect of prolonged periods of rest and inactivity that are typical of many people's lives. You only have to think of how a leg looks after being immobilised in plaster for six weeks to realise exactly what is happening to the whole body of many inactive people as they grow older.

Think now of any active, older person you know. Active people look better, feel better and have more energy, vitality and fun. We all know the feeling of getting back to full strength after illness or injury and its subsequent inactivity – that moment when fatigue lifts and we are rewarded with a surge of energy and exhilaration. This is what activity can do for our bodies and for our lives.

Living actively

Inactivity, not ageing, is the enemy. When we become prematurely fatter, shorter, weaker, sicker and more dependent, much of this is due to activity levels that fall far below safe thresholds for health. Living actively will ensure that our bodies are leaner, taller, stronger and healthier. Our Body Age will be less than our years and we will look and feel good, increase our quality and length of life.

It doesn't even matter if we have never been fit and active previously. At every age our bodies will respond to activity by getting stronger. Almost as soon as we begin we will feel the benefit, and within weeks we will see the benefits in our performance of daily tasks.

Active Living means different things to each of us. Some people will prefer putting extra activity into everyday tasks: walking to the shops more briskly, doing more gardening, even running up and down the stairs 10 extra times a day. Others will prefer a regular or recreational activity – formal exercise sessions at home or in a class with an instructor. Many of us will prefer a combination of all these. The important thing is to decide what is right for you and ... to begin!

The Fitness For Life journey

Think of Fitness For Life as a journey of exploration. It investigates fitness, activity and ageing. It gives clear guidelines on safe, effective and realistic exercise programming, and surprises with just how little you have to do to enjoy health benefits. The Fitness for Life Exercise Plan is safe, successful and progressive; strengthening muscles and bones, improving stamina, co-ordination, balance and flexibility, whether you opt for a challenge or a more gentle workout in a chair. There is also an Exercise Essentials (see Chapter 5) section that reveals the rejuvenating secrets of good posture. Most of all, it is attuned to our daily lives.

Modern living has created a life of too much ease, and while we don't want to put back the daily grind, we do need to be more active. This gives us the best of both worlds and makes ageing a time of vitality, enjoyment, leisure and fulfilment. Fitness For Life is an invitation to begin today and to make a life-long commitment to being more active, more often, for longer.

1

The case for exercise

Fitness is the ability to do what we reasonably want to with our body, in a physical sense. Whatever our age, we want to be able to walk, move, or lift as much as is appropriate to our needs of the moment, in work, shopping, looking after children, taking out the dog, gardening, or travelling. We may also want to participate in a sport at a recreational or competitive level. Health, on the other hand, is an absence of illness or disease. So, although fitness and health are different qualities, they are two sides of the same coin, as physical fitness is central to health.

However, it is possible (and very common) to be healthy but unfit, that is, many people have no disease of any kind, but are too unfit to walk any distance without tiring. Incidentally, we can be fairly fat yet pretty fit – and we can also be slim but very unfit – physical appearances can be deceptive!

It is also a fact that some people are simply born very much fitter than others. Were we to take a hundred 20-year-old untrained men or women of exactly the same weight and size, and test any of the major components of fitness, described below, the range of fitness levels would be so great that those in the bottom quarter could train daily for a year and still not come near the levels that those in the top quarter start with. We would get a similar range of variation with 60-year-olds, but this time the reason would probably have more to do with lifestyle than with natural fitness levels.

Keep active and stay fit

Luckily, in terms of health-related fitness in later life, it is how active we are rather than how fit we are (in sport or laboratory terms) which counts. The more active we are, the fitter we remain. Activity involves physical exercise, which means just about any physical activity which uses our muscles. It includes walking, going up or down stairs, housework, cleaning the car, gardening, or playing with children. It also includes dance in all its forms, all types of aerobics and exercise classes, and almost every sport.

As we get older, fitness and health gradually come closer together. The phrase 'if we don't use it, we lose it', is extremely relevant once we get past 50, but probably also from our mid-thirties. Much of the gradual failure in physical powers is simply due to lack of use – what athletes call 'detraining'. If the detraining process goes far enough, eventually we may not be able to walk as far as we want, or go up hills, or easily bend, or lift as much as we would like.

This is because inactivity leads to a poor heart and circulation, weaker muscles, thinner bones, less flexible joints, more fat, slower reflexes and a greater liability to many illnesses, including heart attacks. This is why, as time goes by, the amount of our general physical activity plays an increasing part in determining how healthy we remain.

What is fitness?

Physical fitness is not a single attribute, but a collection of factors, as follows:

1 Aerobic fitness which involves the lungs, heart and blood-vessels in delivering oxygen and fuels in the blood to release energy in the working muscles; as in distance running, cycling, swimming, jogging, walking, shopping or playing in the park with children. It helps to control heart disease and related circulatory problems.

2 Anaerobic fitness (or local muscle endurance) which involves the muscles themselves working especially hard. Normally, when we work 'within ourselves' the energy is released in muscle with the aid of oxygen. When we move faster, we have to supply more oxygen, until there comes a time when our heart is supplying oxygen to our muscles as fast as it can. If we want to go faster still, then another non-oxygen – or 'anaerobic' – energy source has to come into action. This lets us work much harder, making repeated muscle contractions but only for short periods without resting. This capacity for constant repetition is referred to as endurance – often called local muscle endurance. We need such 'anaerobic fitness' when we go up stairs fast, hurry to catch a bus, or carry a heavy case. (In sport, it is needed in 400-metre running, or rowing; or in gymnastics on the rings or parallel bars.) Oddly, anaerobic fitness is possibly the fitness prerequisite which deteriorates least, because we use it frequently in everyday movements. The other factors that make up muscle fitness are strength, speed and flexibility.

3 Muscle strength This is the force which muscles develop. A reasonable amount of strength is important in life, for carrying shopping or luggage or children, or moving the wardrobe. Especially as we get older, maintaining grip strength is important for unscrewing the tops of jars or bottles, or even opening plastic wraps. Leg strength is important for getting out of armchairs, and arm strength is needed to get on buses, while strength in both is needed to get out of the bath! Strength is also an important requirement of many sports.

4 Muscle speed In everyday life, speed is the least important of the fitness attributes, and it is often bound up with our 'reaction time'. Nevertheless, muscle speed is very useful to catch or deflect household items before they hit the floor, or make a short, quick run for a bus. Of course, speed is important in a whole range of sports.

5 Flexibility is the range of movement at a joint, and is important in everyday life for many tasks, including tying shoe laces, dressing, scratching your back, doing up zips, and putting luggage on racks in public transport. In sport, flexibility is especially important to help prevent pulled or torn muscles.

6 Body composition The percentage amount of fat in our body is also very important. We should keep our body fat in moderation, as there is a level of 'essential body fat' below which it is exceedingly unhealthy for anyone to go. In women, a little plumpness is associated with less thinning of bone.

A reasonable target is to keep our weight to no more than one to two stones (6.5 to 13 kg) heavier than when we left school. It is considered 'normal' to gradually put on weight throughout life, although most of us, through inactivity, gradually lose muscle as we get older, so we should not go on getting heavier! Being much too fat is a major health hazard, increasing the

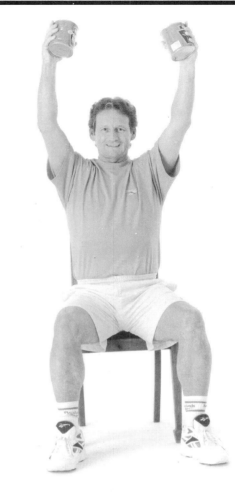

Muscle strength/muscle endurance in the kitchen!

likelihood of heart attack, high blood pressure, diabetes, and joint and circulation problems. However, the good news is that fat can be regulated through eating a bit less and exercising a bit more, but over months or years, rather than the days or weeks of so called 'crash diets', which are almost invariably self-defeating.

7 Motor skills These include factors such as agility, balance, reaction-times and co-ordination, and are harder to measure than the other six. Nevertheless, sport, exercise and activity in general do

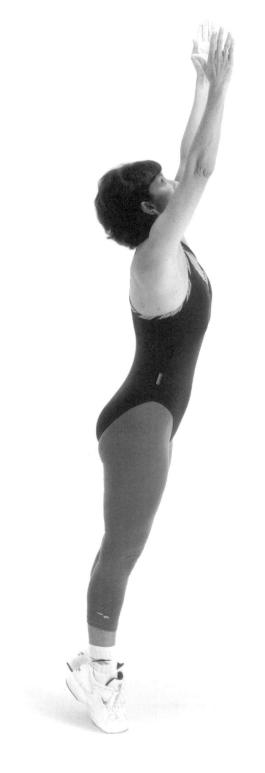

This is fitness.

increase some of these factors. For example, when we exercise or otherwise increase our activity, our balance often improves; and we may lessen the gradual deterioration in our reaction and movement times.

While the first five items above are the main components of physical fitness, all seven are important when we are older, either for health reasons or to ensure a better lifestyle – making daily tasks easier, and letting us remain mobile and independent.

Health problems caused by inactivity

An inactive lifestyle is a far greater threat to health than the processes of ageing, and inactivity is a risk factor that increases with age; a habit that is as serious as smoking in terms of some of the risk factors. Conditions such as obesity, diabetes, stroke, high blood pressure, coronary heart disease, osteoporosis, loss of flexibility, loss of activity of the immune system, chronic fatigue and mental depression are closely associated with a sedentary lifestyle.

Note that we do not have to 'exercise' formally or participate in a sport in order to be active. Activity includes walking to and from the shops or work, work itself, dancing, exercising a dog, playing with children, or climbing stairs or a hill. However, specific exercise such as aerobics classes or swimming, or organised sports such as golf, cricket, tennis, squash or bowls, are often more enjoyable ways to be active, with social benefits as a bonus. But activity itself is the vital factor. Our muscles, heart and joints do not know which we are doing – they simply respond to (and benefit from) the physical demands.

Benefits of regular exercise

Regular exercise has measurable benefits. For example, Dr Darrell Menard (sports scientist) reported a study on two groups of 15 men studied over 23 years. One group took part in regular aerobic exercise, while the other group took no regular exercise. Some of the results were:

1 The exercisers had an average of a healthy 15.9 per cent body fat, compared to the other group's rather fat (for men) 25.7 per cent.

2 The resting pulse rate of the exercisers averaged 10 beats/min lower, and their maximum heart rate was 20 beats/min higher, that is, the active group had much better functional reserves in their heart, and their average blood pressure was healthily lower.

3 The aerobic fitness level of the inactive group had declined by 41 per cent, but that of the active group had gone down only 13 per cent over the 23 years.

Clearly then, being reasonably active can make a great difference to both your health and your lifestyle. Among the main trends which people worry about in terms of ageing are: getting shorter, becoming round-shouldered, getting thinner bones, becoming too fat, developing incontinence, becoming weaker and unsteady, and becoming short of breath. As we will see, even quite modest activity may help to ameliorate these conditions.

Let's preview some of the main benefits to health and general well-being associated with regular activity. Many of these will be discussed in greater detail in Chapter 2.

With regular activity

1 **The heart and lungs** Heart function improves, which lessens the effects of chronic disease, including coronary heart disease. The heart becomes more 'electrically stable', which lessens the risk of heart attack. Blood pressure is reduced, which helps those with mild hypertension, and reduces the 'normal' age-related rise in blood pressure. Blood circulation is improved, which, for example, helps to reduce ankle swelling, leg ulcers, and even chilblains. Some forms of asthma are improved by exercise.

2 **Muscles** Regular activity improves the capacity of muscle to produce both aerobic and anaerobic energy. It also improves the blood supply to the muscle fibres by considerably increasing the network of tiny muscle capillary blood vessels. And, of especial value in later life, activity strengthens the working muscles, and may help with better posture and to ease incontinence. It also increases strength and endurance, and reduces fatigue and the rate of injuries from falls.

3 **Joints and tendons** Activity improves the internal lubrication and nutrition of joints, as well as maintaining flexibility. This reduces the risk of injury, and it may help limit the effects of degenerative arthritis. Frequent activity strengthens tendons and ligaments, and maintains their elasticity. This helps with balance and increases the stability of joints, especially of the knees and ankles.

4 Bones and skeleton Frequent weight-bearing activity helps prevent serious loss of calcium from the bones, allowing them to retain their density and thickness for much longer. Exercise may also help to keep the backbone straight, help minimise back pain and reduce the risk of fracture.

5 Brain, nerve and psychology From the time we are born we lose brain and nerve cells, a loss which may be modified by exercise. Exercise also improves mood, confidence and reaction times.

6 Metabolic functions Regular exercise greatly assists in the control of body weight, by regulating appetite and improving the metabolism of fat. It also helps to prevent 'late-onset diabetes' by making insulin more effective; and it helps the immune system to function better, which may lessen our chances of getting a chest infection, or even some tumours.

Growing old disgracefully

With life expectation ever increasing, it makes sense to remain active, thus preserving strength and power for everyday actions and maintaining, even improving, our quality of life. We can be stronger, leaner, taller, healthier, or managing illness better than our sedentary counterparts, and we can enjoy a good level of mobility, independence and a longer life.

The point of Fitness for Life is that we can take responsibility for our own lives. There is so much we can do. Muscles can and do grow stronger at any age, bones become denser; posture, body shape and balance improves, breathlessness disappears and we gain confidence, energy and a rejuvenating vitality that makes the years drop away – by remaining active.

Dispelling the exercise ageing myths

Myths have a way of becoming fiercely held beliefs that strongly shape our actions or, in this case, lack of action! Fortunately, great advances have been made in the science of exercise and the art of ageing in recent years. And the good news is that there's lots of good news!

HOW OLD IS 'OLD'?

The definition of an 'older person' varies not only according to place but also time. 'Elderly', once described people over 65, but now defines those over 75. Much as we dislike being categorised, it helps to have an idea of when to expect shades of change to take place. Even though it is Body Age, not actual age, that counts.

A recent, sensible set of definitions by gerontologists re-draws the age boundaries.

50 to 65	Mature
65 to 75	Senior
75 to 90	Elderly
90 to 115	Aged

The reason for these new definitions is the population explosion in the older generation, which now spans an age range of more than 40 years. At present, women outnumber men by three to one. It is projected, however, that by the year 2026 older women will outnumber men by two to one. We are all living longer, and by the year 2000 the over 65 group will account for 30 per cent of the population. It will be a powerful economic and social force.

'I am too old to exercise; it's too late for me', or 'It's all right for you, you're young.'

FALSE

On the contrary, if we are over 25 we are too old *not* to exercise!

Many people assume that loss of strength, puffing on mild exertion, stiffness and weight gain are an inevitable part of growing older, when in fact they are often the results of increasing inactivity and loss of fitness. Fitness tends to be wrongly associated only with vigorous competitive sport and the super athlete, rather than with the lives of ordinary men and women. Studies have shown that for healthy, but seriously inactive older persons, even dressing can be such hard work that it may take hours to recover. Without fitness they have become old before their time. Yet it need not have happened. Regular exercise and active living keep the body younger than its years.

'I am very fit for my age' is something we often hear from relatively inactive people and as long as we continue to think in terms of actual age, as opposed to Body Age, our expectations will always be low. If these same people became more active, then they would be amazed at the difference.

It is also important to remember that fitness cannot be stored in the body. Older people often feel they must be fit because they played tennis every day in their twenties and thirties and speak of it as though it were yesterday. Muscle begins to waste after a few days of inactivity, and aerobic fitness begins to be lost after two or three weeks.

So fitness is simple: 'Use it or lose it.' It depends not on your past but on your present amount of activity. The good news is that the older people we work with say they feel fitter than they've ever felt and years younger.

'Older muscle responds to training by getting stronger, leaner and more pliable'

TRUE

Although our muscles are less strong and muscle fibres become smaller as we age, in percentage terms each remaining muscle fibre shows the same potential to improve as younger muscle. In one study at London's Royal Free Hospital Medical School Human Performance Laboratory, women aged 75 to 93, training three times a week for 12 weeks, increased their strength by 24 to 30 per cent.

If we can make our muscle fibres sufficiently strong so that we use fewer fibres to carry out the same task, we will be less tired and conserve energy.

'Weight training is one of the safest, most efficient ways to improve posture and performance of daily tasks – at any age.'

TRUE

Not to be confused with the Olympic sport of weight lifting, weight training, sometimes known as strength training, is a less extreme method of increasing our strength. This can be done in a fitness gym but it also happens in the kitchen; every time we lift a full kettle or a pan of potatoes we are weight training!

The weight training in this book is a steadily progressed 'whole body' muscle conditioning method that puts just the right amount of stress on the muscles i.e., a little more than our muscles are used to, but not too much. This will be different for each of us, and different for various parts of our bodies. The weight of the 'weight' is important. The idea is to find the weight at which you feel comfortable but challenged. To start with, just lifting an arm may be sufficient challenge. When this is done regularly the muscle adapts by getting stronger and you are then ready to progress to the next level.

In the past, studies with older people never progressed beyond very light weights: 4oz or 8oz (100 or 225g) maximum. A bag of flour may be about six times heavier! Studies have shown that to see increases in strength and bone, we need to work using heavier weights. With correct technique we can safeguard the joints.

'Women who work with weights develop big, unsightly muscles.'

FALSE

Many women miss out on the health-giving benefits of weight training because of this myth. Yet women need such training even more because of the effects of the menopause on bone density. Women's hormonal make-up differs from men's; lower testosterone levels mean that women simply cannot develop huge muscles. Instead, the tone and shape of the body looks and feels firmer, and the bones become thicker and less prone to fracture.

'Weight training can help with weight control.'

TRUE

Many people are put off weight training, or even exercise, because they fear that their body fat will 'turn into muscle' if they don't lose weight first. They also worry that if they then stop exercising their muscles will 'turn to fat.' Fat and muscle are two completely different tissues; muscle is an active tissue with a nerve and blood supply, fat is an inert fuel storage depot. Turning fat into muscle would be like trying to turn apples into oranges. Only too much food can be laid down as fat! It is worth remembering though, that soft muscle feels like fat.

Weight control is primarily about fat loss. A little fat is important; too much fat is a high risk to our health. Weight control is about balancing our energy input (the foods we eat), and our energy output (the energy we expend in daily living). Energy is measured in calories; successful weight control involves manipulating the energy balance so that the number of calories expended equals the number of calories eaten. Then the energy stores in the body are neither depleted nor overloaded. Every type of physical activity burns calories and this aids fat loss. The amount lost will depend on how long, how hard, and how often the activity is performed.

Regular activity also makes stronger, leaner muscles. We may, however, see a slight increase in weight, even though we feel and look trimmer. This is because muscle is heavier than fat. However, muscle is metabolically active tissue and, even at rest, burns more calories. Exercise is also known to have an after burner effect whereby calorie burning goes on for several hours after the exercise has ceased. Dieting, on the other hand, often results in loss of muscle as well as fat; yet it is muscle that gives us shape and firmness, and helps in weight control.

'I can spot-reduce fat.'

FALSE!

It is impossible to lose fat from specific areas simply by doing muscular conditioning exercises for those areas. Fat is lost from all over the body and the most effective combination is aerobic and muscle conditioning activities, such as brisk walking and weight training, plus following a sensible eating plan.

'Everything in moderation.'

TRUE AND DOUBLE TRUE!

This timeless truth is the perfect guide to activity for health. The notions 'no pain, no gain' and 'going for the burn' that promoted hard exercise have been thoroughly discredited. Pain is a warning that something is wrong and medical advice must be sought. It is, however, important to distinguish between discomfort and pain. Your muscles may feel a little sore at the beginning but discomfort is not pain. The Fitness for Life Safety Guidelines (see pages 33-5) will teach you how to listen to your body, read its signs and adjust your exercise accordingly. The workout is designed in a particular order to avoid or minimise muscle stiffness.

We don't have to be Olympic material to be fit. Active living is all we need to gain the health benefits of fitness. 'Light active living', with activities such as gardening and walking that add up to 30 minutes per day, is enough to have a healthier heart. The real rewards however, are to be found if we can go that little bit further and build up to 'moderate active living', 30 to 40 minutes of regular, consecutive, brisker exercise such as walking.

'But I've always done it this way and it's never done me any harm.'

FALSE

Keeping up with the times is very important. Science has added much to today's exercise plans. Great attention is paid to back, neck and general joint care, to prevention of wear and tear, injury and fatigue. A more measured pace of performance allows for better technique and control of movement, and there is greater emphasis on the relation of the exercise to posture and to life. Once we have mastered the exercises and new skills, we can feel confident that they not only feel good, but are doing us good too.

'A little of what you fancy does you good!'

TRUE

This is the most fundamental Fitness Fact. We need to enjoy it or we won't do it for long! We each need to discover an activity, or combination of activities, that is stimulating and enjoyable. Keeping an open mind, and reviewing our active living combinations regularly will ensure that we get the best from them.

Active Living and the fitness it brings will enable us to live life to the full. Rest is vital for repair but it is **activity** that rejuvenates.

We now need to consider the facts of ageing, and the changes that occur, so we can be aware of just how essential activity is for a healthy, independent old age.

CHAPTER 2

The inside story

Many of the changes that were once attributed to the ageing process are now known to be due to disease, environmental influences and, particularly, physical inactivity. In general, ageing is not a process with a sudden onset at 40 or 50, or 60; rather it is a process of slow onset that begins in the womb, and continues throughout our life's span. The changes cannot be wholly avoided, but to a considerable extent their effects can be postponed.

The lungs and the heart

Nowhere are the above statements better illustrated than in the case of the lungs and heart, and what makes up the whole 'aerobic system'.

The function of the **lungs** is to act as a bellows, and to suck in and expel air – about 10 litres (just over two gallons) of air per minute at rest, from which about a quarter of a litre of oxygen is extracted. During strenuous exercise, over 100 litres of air may be breathed in and out, with an uptake of over five litres of oxygen and the release of roughly similar amounts of carbon dioxide.

The function of the **heart** is to act as a muscular pump, indeed it is really two pumps side-by-side; one pumping blood to the lungs, and the other supplying the body, both at five litres per minute at rest. During exercise both these rates may be increased three to five times.

The effect of the lungs and heart acting together is seen particularly in 'aerobic' (with air) exercise. One very common aerobic sport is marathon running (26 miles), which serves as a good example to quantify age changes in aerobic function. In their twenties and thirties, top class men will run it in about 2h 15m, and women about 2h 35m. Equivalent men in their sixties will take under three hours, and will break four hours in their seventies, with women taking under four hours in their sixties and breaking five hours right through their seventies.

Few of us can aspire to such performances (below), but the point of these examples is that they show what can be done. Much of the ageing problem in performance is due to the lack of activity which often accompanies ageing, rather than the age process itself. Nevertheless, there is a decline in the various human aerobic functional capacities and physiological measurements.

Age-related changes

By the age of 70, the largest breath size which we can take has fallen by some 40 per cent. However, we actually have so much lung tissue, that healthy lungs are not a limiting factor to the sort of exercise we suggest.

A noticeable change in the respiratory system is that the brain's 'respiratory centre' for controlling breathing becomes more sensi-

tive to the carbon dioxide which the muscles and other tissues give off. This means that when you are older you get a bit more breathless for the same effort, so you feel a bit less fit than you really are.

Similarly, the heart and blood vessels show signs of slow but progressive functional deterioration. The first gradual change is a reduction in the amount of blood the heart can pump in a minute. Partly, this is due to a gradual drop in the maximum heart rate, by some 50 beats per minute between the ages of 20 and 70. Don't be depressed about this – the vast majority of people are entirely unaware that it happens! Very approximately, your maximum heart rate is the figure 220 minus your age. So a 60-year-old will usually have a maximum heart rate of 220 – 60 = 160. This is just a general rule; there are many exceptions. Nevertheless, the rule does provide a rough working guide for those who may like to jog or walk at a set percentage of their maximum heart rate.

As it gets older, the heart takes slightly longer to return to its resting rate after exercise. This is only important in veteran athletes and others who like to do interval training based on time (rather than heart rate). A 'two-minute work, one-minute rest' schedule for a 30-year-old may well need to be modified to 'one-minute work, two-minutes (or longer) rest' 20 years later. Nevertheless, the heart is still capable of improvement, at virtually any age, and you may not experience much of a drop in heart function at all.

In the laboratory, the whole of aerobic fitness can be summed up in two findings, the Maximum Oxygen Intake ('$\dot{V}O_2max$') and the Anaerobic Threshold. The first is an indication of the maximum rate at which the body (mainly its muscles) can use oxygen, and the

AGE DEFYING PERFORMANCES

An 86-year-old man has run the marathon in 5h 40m 12s – an average of 12m 58s per mile. An 83-year-old woman has run it in 4h 52m 36s, an average of 11m 09s per mile. In 1974, a 98-year-old Greek man finished a marathon in 7h 33m. The last of the 25,000 finishers in the London marathon took just over 9 hours.

Aged 41, Jack Foster of New Zealand ran the marathon in 2h 11m 19s.

Aged 42, Priscilla Welch ran 2h 26m 51s. At 40, Eamonn Coghlan ran the mile in under 4 minutes. At 42, Yekaterina Podkopayeva ran 1500 metres in under 4 minutes; she missed winning the European 1500 metres championship by less than half a second.

second is the percentage of that $\dot{V}O_2$max which can be maintained for a reasonable length of time – from 30 minutes to several hours. The 'normal' $\dot{V}O_2$max in the 20s age group is about 45ml/kg/min for men, and just under 40 for women. These values drop by about 5ml/kg/min per decade after about 35 in both sexes, in other words, there is a fall-off of roughly 10 to 15 per cent per decade in aerobic function.

The main question is: 'What proportion of this fitness fall-off is due to the processes of ageing itself, and what proportion to the progressive lack of physical activity which usually accompanies ageing?' Almost all of us, for whatever reason, simply become less physically active the older we get. A very rough answer might be that half of the decline in aerobic fitness is due to the age changes themselves, but that half of the decline is due to physical inactivity – and that can be under our control.

The heartening news is that your aerobic function is still capable of considerable improvement at virtually any age.

Older subjects have been shown not only to increase their aerobic capacity but also to be able to continue to use a higher percentage of it (because they had raised their 'anaerobic threshold'). This is especially useful in such activities as swimming, cycling, aerobics and country dancing, to say nothing of easing the burden of walking (especially on hilly streets and against the wind), shopping, gardening and travelling.

The muscles

Muscle is a tissue whose only ability is to develop a force. It does this because, in each of its cells (often called 'fibres') there are enormous numbers of regularly arranged 'sarcomeres', which shorten and actually develop the force.

Muscle can use its force in three main ways:

1 It can generate a short-term strong movement as in lifting something very heavy, such as a suitcase.

2 It can make a very fast movement, as when we try to catch something falling off a table.

3 It can make repeated movements over a relatively long time, as the leg muscles do in walking, jogging, cycling or dancing, or the arm muscles do in polishing, sweeping, ironing or digging. So, the muscle can be said to show strength, speed and local muscle endurance. Where speed also involves strength, the muscle also develops power; that is, fast strength.

Here are a few more facts about muscle that are of interest to anyone embarking on an exercise programme.

✦ Muscle can generate the energy for its work either by using oxygen to extract the chemical energy from the food – 'aerobic work'; or it can generate the energy from the food without oxygen, for about 30 seconds 'anaerobic work' (which is associated with the rapid onset of fatigue, as in climbing stairs fast).

✦ We have two types of muscle cell: 'slow' and 'fast'. The slow fibres work mainly aerobically, and have excellent endurance. The fast fibres contract about twice as fast, work mainly anaerobically, and have poor endurance. Most of us have about half of each type, but some have very high proportions of fast fibres. Such people look 'muscular', and are generally fast and strong. Others have very high proportions of slow fibres, which gives them a lean appearance, and an excellence at aerobic endurance, as in long distance events.

✦ Muscle fibres are stimulated by nerve fibres, ultimately from the brain. Each nerve fibre controls a number of muscle fibres. Each muscle fibre has between about two and eight capillary blood vessels around it. These bring in the necessary glucose and fat for fuel; amino-acids for building; vitamins, minerals and hormones for function, and oxygen for releasing aerobic energy. They also remove waste products, including carbon dioxide from aerobic work and lactic acid from anaerobic work, as well as, very important, removing heat. We know how hot we can get through muscular work such as heavy gardening.

Age-related changes in muscle

The problem with investigating these changes is that ageing is often associated with increasing inactivity. And both produce similar effects. For example, when a young person's muscle is immobilised in a plaster cast for a bone fracture, many of the changes normally attributable to ageing occur.

The muscle fibres do not change much with age, up to at least 65. There is some atrophy or 'shrinkage', of the fibres, and of the whole muscle. To some degree however, in many older people, this may be masked by an increase in the amount of fat stored around the muscle.

Static (isometric) strength is used when little movement is expected, although a lot of force may be exerted, as in moving the washing machine, or unscrewing bottle tops. From about the mid-twenties, isometric strength begins to deteriorate slowly in both sexes – although there is little noticeable fall-off in strength until the mid-forties, when there is about a 25 per cent fall-off until 65. In women there is an extra fall-off at the menopause. Professor Archie Young, for example, has noted that, especially from the age of about 65 onwards, power (fast strength) is lost much quicker than simple strength (the ability to produce force). He found that, from 65, power declines at a rate of about 3.5 per cent per year, compared to 1.8 per cent per year for strength. Also, the ability to lift things up (concentric strength) is lost more rapidly than the ability to resist a pull on the muscles, as in laying something down (eccentric strength). Finally, as we age, local muscle endurance seems to be maintained better than strength.

Good news from research

There is some very heartening research, showing that the ability of ageing muscle to respond to the training effects of exercise is not lost. Professor Bengt Saltin (one of the world's leading exercise physiologists, working in the Karolinska Institute in Stockholm) has noted that older subjects who continued to train for strength, showed isometric and general strength, speed of movement, and cross-sectional muscle area *identical* to young control subjects. This led him to suggest that 'strength training can counteract the age-related changes in function of the ageing human skeletal muscle'. Similarly, work from the University of Jyvaskyla in Finland on the effects of eight weeks' endurance training on the muscle of 56 to 70 year-old-men, showed that both aerobic and anaerobic muscle function increased. 'The effects of training were *similar* to those previously reported for younger men.' Very recently, Lee Chin Yong, a 69-year-old South Korean estate agent broke the world age record for chin-ups by hoisting himself to the bar 612 times, beating his own record of a year earlier by 242. An extraordinary example of local muscle endurance.

In still another study, it has been found that ageing-but-trained runners had *similar* numbers of capillary blood vessels per square millimetre of muscle to young runners of the same ability (388 compared to 367), although not as many as elite young runners (444).

In perhaps the most cheering study of all, Dr Maria Fiataroni (a medically qualified sports scientist, especially interested in the changes produced in older people by training) devised strength training programmes for a hospital group in their nineties, and in some cases they doubled the strength of their thigh muscles. In only eight weeks on a (relatively) high-intensity progressive resistance programme, they increased their quadriceps strength from an average of 7.6kg to 19.3kg. This meant that some were then able to walk unaided, whereas previously they had been unable to do so. But more particularly, it emphasised the sheer trainability of human muscle. In elderly people this can be very important in terms of their life style. It can enable them, for example, to get in and out of the bath unaided, up from a toilet seat, and onto a bus safely. It can increase balance, thus preventing falls, which in view of diminished bone strength, may be very serious.

Finally, we come to those very important muscles of the 'pelvic floor'. These form an effective muscular sling that supports and helps keep the pelvic organs (e.g. bladder, rectum and womb) in position. One of the 'sling's' important functions is to assist in closing the urethra which empties urine out of the bladder. Another is to help close the rectum. One consequence of ageing (and pregnancy and childbirth) is sometimes a degree of incontinence in one or both of these functions. This can be embarrassing, and is much more common than people realise, because nobody talks about it. Prevention or treatment may be greatly helped by strengthening exercises for the muscles of the pelvic floor (see page 63). This goes for men as well as women. A final incentive is that it improves sex life too.

Thus the general message is that although various muscle functions gradually decline with age, most of the changes are reversible to a very worthwhile extent.

Responses to heat and cold

About 70 per cent of the energy which muscles produce comes off as heat, so we get hot with exercise, and have to regulate our body heat. On the other hand, when we are sitting in a cold room, we may lose more heat than we are producing, and become too cold for comfort. Either way, the body attempts to regulate the amount of heat lost, either by glowing red and sweating (to remove it), or by going pale and shivering (to conserve it).

Older people often have poor heat regulation in the cold and may be prone to 'hypothermia'. A combination of lower muscle mass and a lower metabolic rate means that they produce less heat. They also have poorer thermal sensation – don't feel the air as being cold or warm as well or as soon as when they were young. Control of skin blood vessels, to regulate heat, is also poorer. These factors lead to a general loss of heat regulation at rest and during exercise.

However, many physiologists believe that responses to heat and cold are much more closely related to the amount of regular physical activity and to physical fitness, than to age, and that regular physical activity may diminish the risk of hypothermia by improving responses to cold. It is also important for older newcomers to our Fitness For Life Plan to realise that shorter work intervals and longer rests are helpful for the first few weeks, by which time the heat regulating mechanisms (for example sweating) should be much more effective.

Joints

Joints are structures where two or more bones contact each other, such as the hinge joints at the elbow, knee, fingers and toes, or the ball and socket-type joints of the hip and shoulder, or complex joints at the wrist and ankle. An important feature of all such joints is that, where bone meets bone, there is an overlying layer of cartilage (rather like the sorbothane material used to cushion impact in sports shoes). With regular use, this cartilage layer is maintained in a healthy state; with disuse it may become thinner and even develop holes or ulcers – which lead to painful joints. There are a number of other causes of such osteo-arthritis, but lack of exercise can be a precipitating factor, and exercise does maintain joint health.

There are discs of cartilage between each of the vertebrae in your neck and back. These do not act as shock absorbers; instead they stabilise the joints and allow some of the back muscles to become one large shock absorber for the vertebral column. A healthy spine allows some 15 times greater shock absorption. Appropriate mobilising, stretching and strengthening exercises for the lower back, and strengthening for the abdomen, may help to prevent and ameliorate back conditions and help to lessen a tendency to 'round-shoulders'. Most people tend to get a bit shorter as they get older, but research has shown that physically active people shrink less.

Another factor concerning joints is their range of movement. It is important for joint health that they are mobilised through their full practical range of movement several times weekly. This involves mobility and flexibility work, which will have very worthwhile benefits. Not only does it make tying our shoe laces much less troublesome, but stowing luggage in plane, train or bus racks is much easier, as indeed is dressing – or even scratching our back! Wearing a shoe with much of a heel may lead to a short calf muscle, with the potential to injure your Achilles tendon, and similarly, sitting for long periods each day leads to short hip flexor muscles, which is one cause of back pain and bent posture.

Tendons

As mentioned above, tendons connect muscle with bone, and transmit the force the muscle produces. They also modify it and store energy like powerful elastic. Ageing reduces this elasticity, making most physical effort harder. Tendon and ligament both consist of long, rope-like molecules of collagen which form cross-links with each other. Exercise keeps collagen 'young' and elastic. Not only does this help in general economy of movement, but also in maintaining the accuracy of movements. Normal balance in standing is based on a lot of fine muscular movements of the legs and back, pulling us appropriately slightly backwards and forwards; some of this is done by elasticity of the tendons. If this elasticity is allowed to diminish, natural balance lessens, and falling becomes more likely.

Skin

It is appropriate to mention skin because damage to it, such as blisters, often occurs over joints. Skin becomes thinner with age, and thus is more likely to blister and is more easily torn on the removal of adhesive tape, so go gently. This need not be at all worrying, provided we make due allowances.

Also, exercising in the sun needs more care. Each year from about the age of 30 onwards, the skin loses about 2 per cent of the cells which make the melanin pigment which protects us against the sun's (or sunbed's) ultra-violet rays. Thus, the older we get, the more susceptible we become to sunburn. Our skin also shows fewer signs of acute inflammation, so sunburn is less visible, and we have to be more careful.

Bones and skeleton

Although bone may seem very solid, it is in many respects like living coral. It is very responsive to its environment, and the main environmental factors for bone – apart from nutrition, minerals (especially calcium) and vitamins – are the forces that it is subjected to.

Muscle moves bones by means of tendons which attach onto bone. Stresses produce electrical effects in the bone, stimulating bone growth. So we find thicker, stronger bones attached to muscles which are frequently used, as in

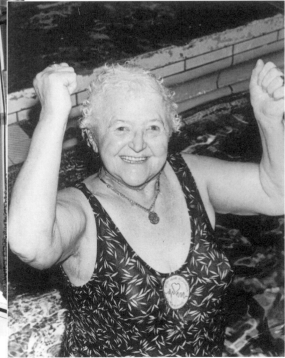

Sail yourself fit, swim yourself fit.

the forearms of professional tennis players. On X-ray, the bone of the racket arm can be seen to be much thicker than in the non-racket arm.

Until about their mid-thirties, men and women increase the thickness or density of their bones, but thereafter bone very slowly loses calcium, and becomes thinner. At the menopause, in response to the marked fall-off of the ovarian hormone oestrogen, women have an accelerated bone loss, especially in the first three post-menopausal years. This leads to a degree of bone thinning or osteoporosis. Osteoporosis is not a disease; it is simply the name given to this thinning of bone. The problem is that osteoporotic bone is more likely to fracture (especially in the hip, spine and wrist). There is a level of bone density which may be said to be the fracture threshold – below this fractures are more likely to occur. This threshold may be pushed back quite considerably by exercise. While older men also have bone loss, they tend to have a bone age of some 15 years younger than equivalent women. The wrist and spine may be affected from our fifties through to our sixties, while the hip usually begins to be affected later. However, we can fight against the effects of osteoporosis by having regular medical checks and ensuring that our diet is adequate – and exercising.

Preventing or delaying bone loss

For best results, the exercise has to be weight-bearing. Brisk walking, jogging, aerobics – especially step-aerobics – country and disco-dancing, and (ropeless) skipping are all recommended. Swimming, cycling and aqua-aerobics are not effective. To some extent, the exercise is site-specific: back raises or back extensions (see page 114) help the vertebrae of the lower back, squats, skipping actions and jogging helps legs and hips, and squeezing tennis balls helps the wrists. There is an important proviso to such exercise: Women already into the fifty plus age range should start such exercise gradually, and stay with these exercises recommended by the Fitness For Life Plan.

Work published at the end of 1994, in the Journal of the American Medical Association, by Dr Miriam Nelson, has suggested that moderate strength training is an effective way to increase bone density. In her 39 subjects, aged from 50 to 70, the 20 who did strength training for 45 minutes twice weekly gained 1 per cent in bone density in their legs and backs over a year, compared to the 19 sedentary controls, who showed a 2.5 per cent fall in bone density – a difference of 3.5 per cent in a single year.

The message is that for both men and women, moderate levels of exercise are very beneficial to bone. Even as late as the age of 80, it appears that exercise may not just slow the rate of bone loss, but may even reverse the trend.

Brain, nerves and psychology

All voluntary skeletal muscle movements start in the brain via nerves down the spinal cord, which then run out to individual motor units in each muscle. The brain itself consists of many thousands of millions of nerve cells. From the time we are in the womb we begin to lose brain cells.

From the mid-forties, the rate of loss of nerve cells increases, such that over the next 35 years the brain decreases about 20 per cent in weight, at a rate of up to 100,000 nerve cells per day. These cells are lost from the cerebral cortex, the spinal cord, and the nerves themselves. Fortunately, the brain has a very large spare capacity!

Nevertheless, neurophysiologists have shown that a 'use it or lose it' principle applies to nerve cells as it does to muscle, in that regular stimulation delays age decay.

With age, there is an increase in the 'central processing' time of reactions, which affects co-ordination. Nevertheless, simple and complex movement times may become faster with training, to such an extent that older, active people may show faster times than sedentary young men and women.

Tremor is often a noticeable aspect of ageing. If we hold our hand out at arm's length, we will probably notice a tremor which is perfectly normal in all of us. Dr Martin Lakie (exercise physiologist at the University of Birmingham, and the British expert on muscle tremor) has noted that through the age range from 10 to 90 years, we have a tremor which becomes slower in frequency but much faster in movement, so it is more obvious and annoying.

A bout of brisk exercise, lasting 20 minutes or so, is also well known to improve mood, and to reduce mild anxiety and depression. This is possibly through the release of morphine-like chemicals in the brain and possibly through the active muscles releasing other brain-influencing chemicals. Indeed, exercise is used as a form of therapy in mild cases of depressive illness.

Finally, it appears that moderate physical exercise programmes improve memory, especially in older age groups. Many studies also show an impressive increase in confidence and improved quality of life.

Metabolic functions

Regular activity greatly assists in the control of body weight by helping to regulate the energy balance of the body, thus preventing obesity-related diseases, including high blood pressure and diabetes. Such activity also helps to regulate appetite, so it may cause the very slim to eat more, and the rather overweight to eat less, as appetite is brought more into line with actual need.

Regular exercise improves the sensitivity of the body to the hormone insulin, which may help to prevent 'late-onset diabetes', which is relatively common in older people.

Exercise also improves fat and 'lipoprotein' metabolism, and prevents blood from clotting too readily, thus helping to prevent disease in the coronary arteries, which may lead to heart attacks.

Finally regarding metabolic effects, as we grow older the immune system gradually functions less effectively. Nevertheless, recent studies suggest that even quite mild exercise may reverse this situation. In China, Dr Sun Xusheng (an exercise scientist at the Shanghai Teachers' University, with an interest in exercise and the immune system) noted, in regular t'ai chi (traditional gentle Chinese exercises) performers over the age of 65, that the number of their 'active T-lymphocytes' increased by 40 per cent. Dr Rajit Chadra (a medical doctor working at the University of Newfoundland, Canada) instituted moderate exercise programmes for three months to a group of his patients aged from 65 to 100 years. He also found improved 'T-lymphocyte' function and that his patients spent an average 40 per cent fewer days in hospital with (mainly) respiratory infections. These 'T-lymphocytes' are very important cells in the immune system, both helping other immune cells and killing virus-infected cells directly.

Thus, light to moderate regular activity or exercise appears to enhance the immune system (in both sexes).

CHAPTER 3

Preparing to exercise

W e hope that what you have read so far has finally convinced you that becoming involved in our Fitness For Life Plan could not only change your life but also extend it. If it has, you will want to start immediately. That's great – but the plan is all about getting you moving effectively and keeping you moving safely, so let's take it a step at a time.

Before you begin on this, or any exercise programme, there are some important checks and preparations that need to be made. If you are prepared to invest the necessary time in this planning stage, you will reap dividends in terms of more enjoyment in your exercise programme, a fitter, healthier body, and an improved life style. Read on!

Your exercise session is one of the most important parts of your day and preparation is half the battle. Give it a high priority.

1. Health screening and fitness assessment

Exercise must be effective to be beneficial but first it must be safe. This means that *before* you do any exercise it is **strongly advisable** to complete the Health Screening Questionnaire on page 31. Take it along to your doctor's surgery, have a full medical examination and secure your doctor's permission to exercise.

The questionnaire will help in assessing your Health Status so that you can be sure of selecting the most beneficial type of exercise programme. And what could be more of a boost than a clean bill of health from your doctor and confirmation of your suitability to exercise?

As we have said, it is not our age but our unique Body Age which counts. No two bodies age at the same rate, so assessing health by guesswork isn't sufficient; simple observation from the outside can be deceptive. It doesn't give us the inside story or take lifestyle factors or family history into account. And these are important. A tick next to ANY of the 16 questions on page 31 means it is essential to have a thorough medical before beginning to exercise.

2. Setting goals

At any age this is the moment of truth. You have decided you definitely want to get fit and to be more active. You feel ready to turn non-action into action as soon as possible. Yet we know this moment is one of the major stumbling blocks that can cause resolve to dwindle and disappear! The cause is almost always the same – we hadn't set any goals. Goal-setting is an important part of preparation.

ASSESSING YOUR BASIC FITNESS LEVEL

Self assessment without testing tends to be very over optimistic, as we have seen from our research. Bearing this in mind and being as honest as possible, assess whether you are fit according to the definitions below, which were used recently in a major national fitness survey. It can be a bit of a shock to be pinned down so closely but this not only enables you to more accurately select the most suitable Fitness for Life Workout Plan to follow, it also gives you a simple baseline from which to chart your future fitness progress. (Record the results and reassess at three and six month intervals.)

✦ If you do three sessions of aerobic activities per week you are fit.

✦ If you do 1 aerobic session per week or do strength or flexibility sessions each week, or have an active lifestyle (e.g. you walk everywhere and do lots of gardening) you are moderately fit.

✦ If you are any less active than the above, you are unfit.

Goals are a statement of intention, they tell us why we are doing something, what is our aim and how long it will take to achieve. It's rather like planning a journey. You know your destination and the routes you can take to get there. It makes all the difference to the experience of travelling if you are confident that you know where you are going, that you will get there in the shortest time possible and that, if there's an emergency, you have an alternative route. Compare this to aimlessly wandering about as so often happens generally in life, and certainly in exercise. Without a goal you probably won't keep going, no matter how enthusiastic you may have been at the beginning.

Set yourself some sensible, achievable goals – both short and long term. They should be personal to you, specific, realistic and measurable. Approach your goal-setting in a practical and effective way; consider the goals that regular exercise can help you fulfil. Then select a time scale, the necessary steps and the activities. Goals need to be up-dated regularly as the goal that got you there won't be the one that keeps you there in the future. It's the striving to achieve, not the actual achievement that will maintain your interest and motivation.

Recent research and experience shows that this first stage can be more difficult for the older person. We may know that 'exercise is good for you' and have the strongest belief in the importance of activity for health of all the age groups, but we are proportionately the least active.

However, once we begin we show a greater commitment, adherence, enthusiasm and sense of fun than any other group of people keeping fit.

Don't be discouraged if you know you

Questionnaire

YES NO

1 Do I get chest pains while at rest and/or during exertion? ☐ ☐

2 If the answer to Question 1 is 'yes', is it true that I haven't had a physician diagnose these pains yet? ☐ ☐

3 Have I ever had a heart attack? ☐ ☐

4 If the answer to Question 3 is 'yes', was my heart attack within the last year? ☐ ☐

5 Do I have high blood pressure? ☐ ☐

6 If you don't know the answer to Question 5, answer this: Was my last blood pressure reading more than 150/100? ☐ ☐

7 Do I have diabetes? ☐ ☐

8 (If the answer to Question 7 is 'yes') Is my diabetes presently going without treatment? ☐ ☐

9 Am I short of breath after extremely mild exertion and sometimes even at rest or at night in bed? ☐ ☐

10 Do I have any ulcerated wounds or cuts on my feet that don't seem to heal? ☐ ☐

11 Have I unexpectedly lost 10 pounds or more in the past 6 months? ☐ ☐

YES NO

12 Do I get pain in my buttocks, the back of my legs, or in my thighs or calves when I walk? ☐ ☐

13 While at rest, do I frequently experience fast irregular heartbeats – or, at the other extreme, very slow beats? (While a low heart rate can be a sign of an efficient and well-conditioned heart, a very low rate can also indicate a cause for concern.) ☐ ☐

14 Am I currently being treated for any heart or circulatory condition, such as vascular disease, stroke, angina, hypertension, congestive heart failure, poor circulation to the legs, valvular heart disease, blood clots, or pulmonary disease? ☐ ☐

15 As an adult, have I ever had a fracture of the hip, spine, or wrist? ☐ ☐

16 Did I have a fall more than twice in the past year (no matter what the reason)? ☐ ☐

Even if you answered 'no' to all 16 questions, you should be aware that the ACSM (American College of Sports Medicine) advise that all people over the age of 35 who are about to begin a physical training programme should ideally have a medical.

Reference: Maria Fiatarone, M.D.
Human Nutrition Center on Aging at
Tufts University, Boston

are quite seriously 'out of shape'. If you are, you probably took quite a long time to get that way. Allow yourself the necessary months for the results of the training to take effect. If you have difficulties, ask for a little help from a friend or, even better, from a qualified fitness professional, to reset your goals and put you back on the road to success.

Finally it is a good idea to record your goals, in a notebook not on a scrap of paper, so that you can measure your progress. And this should be signed and dated. It will help you to be really committed! It may sound a little extreme but it works.

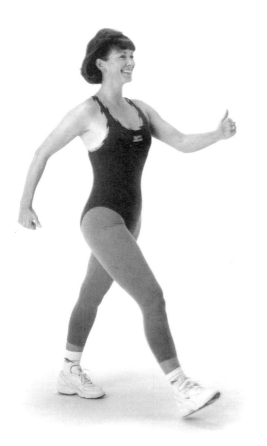

Keeping fit is fun!

3. Selecting a suitable time.

Selecting a time of day that suits you and fits in with your life is one of the great secrets of fitness success. Ask yourself these simple questions. Are you a morning, afternoon or evening person? When is your time your own or, at least, at its quietest?

Also, try to link your exercise time with a daily activity e.g. if you are a morning person try choosing a time before or after doing your teeth or getting dressed. If the evening is your time, try to fit it in before settling in too cosily e.g. exercise before or after watching the news, or feeding the cat. And remember it's always good psychology to build in a reward e.g. before your favourite TV programme or going out. If you are on any medication, especially for joint problems, finding a time when you are at your most mobile and least drowsy, can make all the difference to enjoying the sessions.

Now decide which days of the week are best and how often you will do each activity; trying to ensure a day's rest between the same activity e.g. walking on Monday, Wednesday, Friday; strengthening exercises on Tuesday and Thursday (see Chapter 6 for options).

You now have time slots and a weekly pattern that feel right for you. We have included an example of a weekly programme on page 66.

4. Making a commitment

Write down the programme where you can see it often. Then you can arrange future diary dates around the exercise sessions and, if need be, change the exercise time for a particular day or simply enjoy a day off. Making sure you won't be interrupted, for example by taking the phone off the hook while exercising, is another effective way of ensuring success. You may even persuade a friend or group of friends to start exercising with you (comparing notes on progress is a great motivator).

5. Preparing your exercise area

Making a 'furniture free' safe space in which to move is a priority. The floor surface is particularly important. Smooth out any ripples in the carpet and check that there is nothing on the floor that could cause you to trip. Also, have cushions, towel, mat, chair, weight and other equipment to be used in position. It breaks the flow and resolve if you have to go off and get something half way through. The room should be warm but well ventilated. It is also a good idea to have a drink of **water** before, during and after exercising; 15 minutes before and then every 15 to 20 minutes or so is a good guide.

If exercising out of doors, work on a soft, smooth surface such as grass.

6. What to wear

Wear comfortable clothing that allows your body to breath and move freely. Wear loose fitting clothing, but avoid anything so baggy from head to toe that you are unable to see, and correct, body alignment. Light, 'giving' cotton trousers that fit snugly around the ankles, or shorts and tee shirts work well, or leotards for those who like them.

Avoid synthetics since they prevent sweat evaporating and can cause overheating. At the same time warmth is important as the older body gets colder more easily without you necessarily being aware of it. Wearing layers of clothing that can be discarded gives the extra protection needed when exercising in colder weather.

Footwear Wearing suitable footwear is particularly important; it provides extra protection and a good grip on the floor or ground. Tennis pumps are fine but it is really worth investing in purpose-designed workout shoes. Go for the lightweight, less expensive range of a well known brand. (Sling backs, stockings, slipperettes and shoes with more than a one inch heel are dangerous.) More sturdy fitness shoes are best outdoors. Finally, keep your workout shoes specifically for exercising – feet 'enjoy' a change!

7. Safety first

Here are some golden guidelines that every exerciser at every age and every stage of fitness would be wise to follow.

Listen to your body Exercise should always be comfortable and achievable. If it isn't, your body is trying to tell you that you are overworking, or that you may have an infection hanging about, or that the particular activity doesn't suit your body. Learning to listen to your body, understand what the various signs mean, and adjust your exercise accordingly is an important safety skill.

Learn to distinguish between working comfortably hard and overworking; between fatigue and exhaustion; between discomfort and pain; when exercising can continue and when it should be stopped.

Signs when exercise can be continued When exercising at a beneficial level, in stamina work your breathing *will* be heavier and your heart *will* beat more quickly. This means simply that your heart is responding to the demands of the muscles and the extra work. Your body will start to feel warmer, joints looser and light sweating may occur. This is called 'overload'. Overload, or feeling comfortably challenged, is an essential part of getting fitter.

Signs of overworking (exercise needs to be adjusted *and* can then continue)

You should feel that you are working hard but only comfortably hard. If you feel out of breath, dizzy, exhausted, heavy limbed, clumsy or starting to trip over your own feet, you are working far too hard for your level of fitness. You are overworking and will want to stop, but don't stop suddenly! Keep moving, but change the pace. Bring it down to a comfortable level, making the arm movements smaller or even stopping them. When your energy returns you can pick up the pace again. If you continue to work at too high a level, exhaustion and injury may result and you will come to associate exercise with distress when in fact you were simply doing too much too soon. Overload in strength training is often experienced as a mild burning, fatigue or aching in the muscles; do one more repetition only, then rest or do a different exercise until refreshed and ready to go again.

Discomfort

Discomfort is something you are most likely to feel in the early days, when mild stiffness is not unusual. However, it can also be a sign that you are pushing a bit too hard for your present level of fitness and need to progress more gradually. Discomfort may also be a sign that your body is out of alignment, so always check this with the instructions and photographs.

Signs when exercise should be stopped

Signs when exercise should be stopped Pain of any sort is a warning sign; never ignore it. Stop immediately if necessary;

otherwise, ease down as gradually as possible to a stop. If the pain continues seek medical advice. If there is no medical problem and the pain reoccurs, change the activity.

Pain during or after exercise may be because you have taken a joint beyond its pain free limit e.g. taking the arm too high with a stiff shoulder, or placing too much weight over a weak knee, then adjust the movement and work within the pain free range. **Never** work through pain.

NOTE: Certain joint and other medical conditions such as arthritis may mean there is a constant, low level of pain. Consult your doctor to get clearance to exercise first and then work cautiously and with control, introducing the exercises one at a time and taking the weight off the affected part as much as possible. Appropriate regular exercise can reduce stiffness, but if it increases the pain, change the activity. If pain has not returned to 'normal' within two hours after exercising, then discontinue the programme and seek medical advice. **Never** exercise a joint that is inflamed, swollen or hot to touch. Rest is what is required.

Health wise, weather wise

At every age it is important to remember that there is no gain where there is pain and strain. Where your body is concerned, be guided by its very good common sense.

✦ Never do any vigorous stamina, strengthening or stretching with an infection or temperature.

✦ Never do any vigorous stamina work after a cold (or any respiratory illness such as bronchitis) for nine days after the symptoms have cleared. A little non-weight-bearing mobility work is fine whatever your health or the weather.

✦ Never do any outdoor exercise in icy, chill factor conditions.

✦ Always reduce the intensity of your exercise in heat and humidity.

✦ Always avoid the risks of falling.

✦ Avoid an over-energetic start.

✦ Avoid trying to beat the clock.

✦ Avoid being over-ambitious.

✦ Remember exercise is not about winning, it's about fitness for health. We cannot over stress the importance of this. Finally, if you are going to attend an exercise session, make sure the teacher is qualified. Similarly, if you intend to use a home video, make sure it is made by exercise and sports science professionals, with the backing of a national body such as the Sports Council.

8. Be flexible in body and mind

Be adaptable and resourceful. If there is not time for your planned workout, just do a warm up (see pages 68–91). If you cannot attend your usual class, go for a walk instead. If it is too hot, go for a swim. Whatever you do, or don't do, it is essential not to worry or feel guilty about missing a session, or even three; just get back into it again as soon as possible. You will be well rewarded by the health and fitness benefits that come your way.

9. Remember, this is fitness for life

It is what we do the majority of the time that counts. Don't let a slip turn into a slide or be an exercise drop out. It's never too late to begin and 'easy does it' is always best.

AND IMMEDIATELY SEEK MEDICAL ADVICE IF YOU EXPERIENCE:

✦ Pain or discomfort in the chest, abdomen, back, neck, jaw or arms.

✦ Dizziness or fainting while you are exercising. (Dizziness can occur if you stop too suddenly after vigorous exercise; this is simply due to insufficient cooling down exercises.)

✦ A nauseous sensation during or after exercise.

✦ Extreme and unfamiliar shortness of breath.

✦ Irregular pulse, skipping a beat.

✦ Very rapid heart rate even after five minutes of rest. (This can often be caused by a fever, tiredness or anxiety but needs to be checked.)

CHAPTER 4

How the programme works

The FITNESS FOR LIFE PLAN has been developed to meet your needs with safety, success and progress in mind. Strengthening muscles and bones, improving stamina, flexibility, co-ordination and balance, the workout can be varied according to the amount of time or energy you have. Better a short, gentle workout than none at all.

The exercises in The Exercise Plan, Chapter 6, are arranged in four sections:
+ Warm-up Exercises
+ Aerobic or Stamina Conditioning Exercises
+ Muscle Conditioning Exercises
  (incorporating Flexibility Stretches)
+ Relaxation and Remobilising Exercises

Every exercise can be done sitting or standing and there are variations to make them more, or less, taxing.

Whenever possible opt for the standing versions as the weight bearing involved helps to strengthen the skeleton. Never, though, risk pushing your body too hard. If, because of joint or other health conditions, you are restricted to the seated options, there are adaptations to add variety and a challenge. Whatever the choice, never be tempted to miss out the warm-up or cool down or consistently miss out one section. Remember, you need all these aspects of fitness.

Each exercise gives detailed instructions to ensure safety, the reasons for doing it, and a description of which joints or muscles are being worked.

The integration of stretches in between

the Muscle Conditioning Exercises is one of the unique features of the Fitness For Life Plan. Unlike other exercise groups, older people do not seem to benefit greatly from a continuous block of stretches, so it is a good idea to incorporate the Cool Down Flexibility Stretches into the Muscle Conditioning section.

Let's look at the Fitness For Life Workout in detail so that you can see where, and how, each part fits into the whole and why you need it. This will help you to make clearer choices about which section to do on certain days. For example on days when you are feeling tense and stressed, an aerobic biased workout would be most beneficial. On other days, the focus of a strength session may be what you need.

The warm-up

The warm-up is an essential part of any activity programme. It gets your body ready to go and focuses your mind on the harder task ahead. It boosts your circulation, creating energy and warmth, which makes muscles more pliable, ligaments more resilient, joints move more freely. It minimises stress on joints, reducing the risks of injury, and greatly improves performance. And the body really does enjoy the activity all the more for a warm-up. If done regularly the warm-up exercises alone will have a rejuvenating effect. The Warm-up is in two parts:

1. Body warming and joint mobilising

Body warming exercises are natural, comfortable, whole body moves such as walking, swinging, marching and dancing. These strongly rhythmical, yet not too

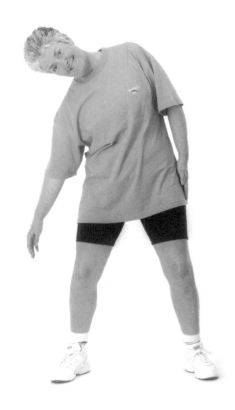

Daily mobility exercises nourish joints

energetic, exercises use the large muscle groups of the arms and legs to get the heart, lungs and circulation going and increase the oxygen rich blood supply to the working muscles. This creates energy and heat, which in turn warms the muscles, making them more resilient and pliable. It also allows your heart beat to increase gradually and steadily maintain a smooth, regular rhythm.

Joint mobilising exercises loosen all the major joints of the body, promoting ease of movement in the spine, shoulders, elbows, wrists, fingers, hips, knees and ankles. They take each joint through its full natural range, with circling, bending, extending moves. Mobilising exercises stimulate the joints' natural lubricant (synovial fluid). This helps to 'oil' and protect the joint, reducing stiffness yet increasing its stability.

The importance of keeping your joints mobile cannot be overemphasised. The most effective mobility work is performed from a stable base, taking each joint or joints slowly and carefully through a full, natural range of movement. When combined with stretching, mobility work will keep joints supple and nourished, maintain correct posture and lengthen the spine.

Ten minutes plus may seem a long time for a warm-up but it is important to take a little longer over this warming process as we get older. The heart and lungs take longer to get going, muscles longer to warm through and joints more thorough preparation.

2. The warm-up stretch

Muscles that have been warmed then stretched slowly and carefully respond better to every demand made of them, be it making the bed, going for a walk, doing a workout or gardening. Pre-stretching the muscles by gently lengthening them also reduces tension, helps to guard against injury in larger, faster moves, and improves posture, poise, and performance.

It is important to stretch all the major muscle groups, the front and back of the legs, chest and back, and the back of the arms, before exercising. Correct alignment is also important; having the foot or leg in the right position can mean the difference between an effective stretch, and a non-effective stretch. Holding the stretch is also important. These warm-up stretches should be held for a count of eight seconds. Natural, regular breathing greatly assists stretching. At any age, stretching can cause injury if we do it when we are cold, or 'bounce' or stretch too strongly.

Older muscles are more vulnerable to injury and shortening, so great care must be taken to stretch correctly. Stretching should always be comfortable and felt in the bulky part of the muscle.

Aerobic or stamina conditioning

The rewards of the Aerobic or Stamina Conditioning Plan (pages 92–101) will be healthy lungs, a powerful heart, a good circulatory system, well conditioned muscles and lots more energy (see page 12).

It consists of steady, rhythmic movements similar to the Body Warmers in the warm-up. Here however, they are larger, more dynamic and performed more vigorously. These exercises are designed to use your body in an increasingly more energetic way so that you have to breathe more deeply. Your heart has to beat a little faster to deliver oxygen to the working muscles. Hence the name 'aerobic' or 'with air'. When this is done regularly your heart and lungs become more efficient and your stamina improves.
The three stages to our Aerobic Workout are:

1. Build-up

The Build-up is when you are gradually increasing your heart rate and body temperature to be ready for the hardest stage. You achieve this by gradually increasing the size of the movement e.g. starting with no arms, then low arms, then larger arm moves and then using the trunk and arms to lift your body to its full height. Similarly your legs begin with small movements and end in large, striding walks, knee lifts and, if enjoyed, small springing or jumping actions.

2. Maintenance

The Maintenance or 'Work' stage is where you have reached a point where you feel you are working hard, yet comfortably hard, so that you can maintain this pace for your 'target' time.

A moderate pace and workload throughout the Maintenance Stage, is essential. Older muscle tends to be slower and fatigues more quickly; faster, more powerful moves are more difficult to sustain without discomfort and exhaustion.

The Fitness For Life Plan maintenance section is designed with this in mind. It achieves a workload that is challenging yet safe by using two well known approaches to physical training:

Interval training plays with intensity or 'effort'; so a moderately energetic move is followed by an interval of more vigorous effort and then returns to the more moderate effort.

Fartlek training, so called after its Swedish namesake, plays with speed or 'pace', so a burst of speedier movement is followed by one that eases the pace. The overall feeling of working hard persists but your body paces itself so that it is always ready to go again. The feeling should always be one of breathing more heavily but never gasping for breath or straining in any way.

These approaches can be applied to every kind of aerobic training, so whether we prefer walking, cycling, swimming, or whatever, we can play with speed and effort to add interest and effectiveness to these activities also. The message is one of moderation. Remember, there is no gain where there is too much strain. Both speed and energy improve with training but not with straining.

The maintenance section also contains some low level 'springing', skipping and jumping actions with good landing and take off technique. This is very strengthening and loads the bones in your hips and lower body. The skill involved in the springing action can greatly improve your balance. It is also the ultimate test for pelvic floor muscles! It is not, however, in any way essential as you can get these benefits in other ways. The Fitness For Life Plan provides other options on every page. So do what suits your body best.

3. Cool down

This is where you gradually ease down your heart rate. Here, you reverse the process of the Build-up by steadily decreasing the size and effort of the moves.

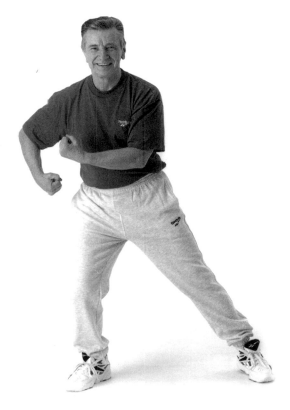

Comfortably challenged

This final phase is particularly important to accommodate the circulatory changes in the older body. To go from working in top gear to a sudden stop may cause you to feel nauseous, dizzy or exhausted. This is all avoidable with a proper 'cool down', which gradually returns your body to a steady state, leaving you refreshed and relaxed. Your heart rate, breathing and body temperature return to the level they were at the end of the warm up. Your blood flow re-routes efficiently back to vital organs and waste products accumulated in your muscles during exercise are removed.

Training without straining

To train without straining, it is important to adjust the Fitness for Life Programme, and all activity, to suit ourselves exactly. Intensity, effort or how hard we are working will be different

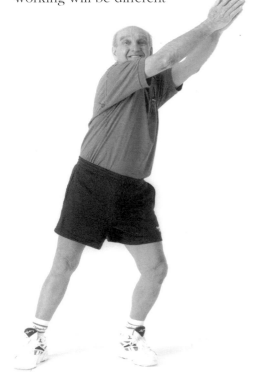

for each of us, and changes as we get fitter. Movements that feel very hard to start with soon become easier.

To increase our fitness we have to 'overload' our heart and lungs. Overload simply means a level of work which is felt as quite vigorous. The fitter we are the harder we have to work to create overload. If you are starting out from a fairly unfit state then 10 minutes at a brisk pace will be enough to create the necessary overload. The less fit you are the easier it is to become fitter.

If you keep the workload challenging but comfortable you will be able to go for longer. If you push too hard for your level of fitness, and are no longer able to sustain the pace, you are no longer working aerobically. You are using 'anaerobic' or shorter lasting stores for releasing energy. You will soon become exhausted and unable to continue. Most movements use combinations of both sorts of energy. When you can sustain a steady effort you are working aerobically, using oxygen to release energy. Working aerobically burns fat for longer and hence is helpful in weight control, and gives you a more streamlined look.

Simple safety measures/ assessing your effort

Whatever your age, it is important to assess your effort by using one of the following safety checks while you are exercising.

Perceived exertion

A good way of assessing your effort is by using a measure of what is termed perceived exertion – in other words, how hard you reckon the exertion is. Gunnar Borg, a Swedish exercise physiologist, developed a scale of perceived exertion ratings. The table below, adapted from the Borg scale, is a sensible, easy-to-use guide to ensure you are working safely. The scale has been tested many times and correlates well with the actual severity of exercise.

As you see, 1 is extremely easy whereas 10 is the hardest level at which you could possibly imagine exercising. If you feel you are exerting yourself at a fairly energetic level, then you might select a rating of perceived exertion (RPE) of 5 or 6. When you reach a level that feels you are working really vigorously, then 7 would probably be right. This is exactly where you want to be. For aerobic work to be safe and effective, the level of perceived exertion should be somewhere between 5 and 7. This scale of self-assessment provides a useful yardstick to ensure you don't get too carried away and equally that you are working hard enough to benefit. Checking the RPE every few minutes ensures that you are training somewhere between 4 and 7, depending on your energy levels that

SCALE OF PERCEIVED EXERTION

0	No exertion at all
1	Just perceptible
2	Extremely light
3	Very light
4	Light
5	Moderate
6	Somewhat hard
7	Hard
8	Very Hard
9	Extremely Hard
10	Maximum exertion

day. It is not recommended that you exceed 7 at any time during the Fitness For Life Plan.

In the Aerobic section aim for between 4 to 5 in the Build-up, 5 to 7 in the Maintenance and 5 to 4 in the Cool Down Aerobics and finally coming down to 4 to 2 before going on to the next part of the workout.

It's hard to believe that something so simple can do the job so well, but it does. When you know the scale off by heart, it becomes second nature and adds interest to the workout.

The Talk Test

Another practical way to ensure you have got the effort right is the Talk Test. You should always be able to carry on a conversation, or even sing. If you find you are gasping for breath, unable to talk, or your legs feel heavy and unco-ordinated, you are working too hard for your present level of fitness. Whenever you need to adjust your exercise effort **do not stop completely**. It is far better to make your arm movements smaller, and ease the pace down a little. Your breathing will ease, your energy will return, and you can continue at a pace that feels right for you on that day.

To ensure maximum effect, put as much effort into each exercise as you can and try to perform the maintenance section with as much energetic enjoyment as you can. If music seems fun, the Aerobic section can be an opportunity to put on your favourites and really let your hair down.

How long and how often?

Ten minutes of moderate activity twice a day is excellent, or five minutes every day will bring some benefits, and even five minutes once a week will bring more than if you do nothing at all! To guarantee even greater health benefits you could work towards achieving the UK Health Education Authority recommendation to aim for 30 minutes of continuous moderate activity five times a week. Then, for the true enthusiast, upping three of these weekly sessions to a more vigorous pace will guarantee optimal health gains.

The world authority, The American College of Sports Medicine (ACSM), states that our aerobic fitness can be gained and maintained, by aiming for thirty minutes of exercise on three days a week, at an intensity of about 5 to 7 on the Borg Scale. At every age this will allow you to enjoy the full health benefits of being aerobically fit.

The length of the **aerobic workout** depends entirely on how fit you are. Three to five minutes is a good place to start. Work up your 'target time' over months, not weeks, increasing the length first and then the pace. Aim to take 12 to 20 weeks to build up to 30 minutes of continuous aerobic activity, always taking three minutes of this time to build up

MODERATION WINS THE DAY

Researchers compared groups of relatively healthy people over a period of 8 years based on their scores on treadmill tests. The fittest worked out long and hard, running as much as 30 to 40 miles a week. The middle groups had active lifestyles that included some formal exercise and the least fit were people who did no formal exercise. The least fit lasted the shortest amount of time on the treadmill and showed a far greater chance of early death from disease; the fittest had life expectancy rates three-and-a-half times higher than the least fit. Yet the most exciting results in improved mortality rates came from the active lifestyle group – people who were only a little more active than the sedentary group **and that's not very far to jump!**

and three or more to wind down.

Even if the target times for either moderate or vigorous aerobic activity sound impossible at the moment, the progressive approach of the Fitness For Life Plan is designed to get you going – at your own pace. It progresses to longer times only when your body is enjoying it so much it is asking for more.

The active living approach

The idea is that you do everything as actively as you possibly can during the course of the day – walking to the post, climbing escalators, carrying the shopping home – timing yourself and aiming to total 30 minutes of such activities each day. We all need simply to be more active, more often, and the more we do the more we will want to do. When you've been exercising in this gentler pattern for a while, and have felt the improvements, the exercise approach suddenly has a greater appeal. It's getting started that's difficult. Use any combination that gets you going. The only thing that matters is that you begin to do something active for your health.

As soon as you can say you are **MORE ACTIVE, MORE OFTEN** you are on your way. Just by circling your shoulders and lengthening your spine to relieve tension you have made a start. Every minute counts towards that activity total, and takes you a step nearer to health benefits.

Even when you are well on your way to doing the recommended number of sessions per week, do continue to live 'actively', as this gives that extra bit of leeway if you have to miss a session.

Remember, the closer you get to the Fitness for Life guidelines, the more benefits you will get, the better you will feel and the longer you are likely to live.

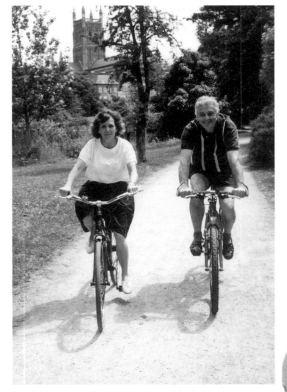

Suggested aerobic activities include cycling
and walking

Aerobic choices for active living

Variety adds spice to our fitness planning.
Consider alternating your Fitness for Life
Aerobic Plan with one or more of the
following. A combination of different
activities will give you even better effects
because you are 'cross training', using a wider
range that relates more to the varied demands
of life. Remember that 'aerobic' exercise does
not mean fast, hard, gruelling and exhausting
but rather moderate, rhythmical and
continuous. Here are some suggested
aerobic activities: walking, cross-country
skiing, swimming, cycling, dancing, rowing,
running, exercising to music, circuit training,
aqua aerobics, skipping. For guidance in
specific activities there is some
recommended reading on page 144.

Muscle conditioning

The Strength, Local Muscular Endurance and Flexibility Training part of the Fitness For Life Plan (see pages 102–135) is, in some ways, the most important in reversing the ageing process. This is because it is designed to train Muscle Fitness. It focuses on training the back, arms and shoulders in the upper body, and the legs, hips, abdominals and pelvic floor in the lower body.

A muscle that is in peak condition is strong, enduring and pliable. The plan uses three types of Muscle Conditioning Exercises: **muscular strength**, **local muscular endurance** (see pages 12–13) and **stretching.**

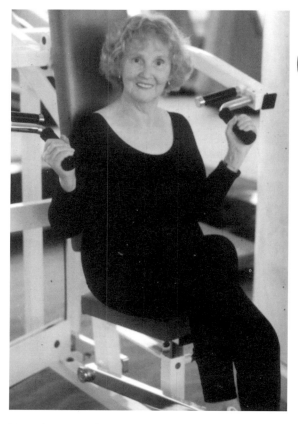

Train those muscles

Muscular strength and local muscular endurance

Muscular Strength is the maximum force we can lift in one go e.g. the holiday suitcases. Local Muscular Endurance is the ability to sustain lighter actions for a prolonged period e.g. washing the windows. We train for strength by lifting heavier weights for a few repetitions. We train for local endurance by lifting lighter weights for more repetitions.

Each muscle can be trained in both ways. **Repetitions** are the number of times we contract the muscles or do the exercise. **Repetition Maximum** is the amount of weight you can lift for a particular number of repetitions, e.g. six repetition maximum is the amount you can lift (with correct technique) for six repetitions, but not for seven or eight. A **set** is a series of repetitions. **Resistance** is an external force against which we can contract the muscles. This could be our own body weight or equipment such as a weight, or both.

What is very hard to start with, and definitely a strength exercise, gradually becomes easier and can be continued for longer and so becomes an endurance exercise once our muscles adapt by becoming stronger. In the Fitness For Life Plan the emphasis is towards strength training because this automatically increases local muscular endurance and because strength is essential to perform everyday tasks. All strength work requires close attention to exercise technique to avoid tension and injury. At any age we must work near to our limit to achieve strength, 'overloading' the muscle, by working with a weight that is a little heavier than we are used to lifting. However, it is wise to begin practising the exercises with little or no weight until you have mastered the correct lifting technique. You can then start with light (e.g. 1lb or 0.5kg) weights, building gradually as you progress towards your strength and endurance goals. (Bags of rice or flour, or cans of food make effective weights.)

To ensure that you get maximum benefit and minimise any risk of injury, the Fitness for Life Plan recommends working along the Strength Endurance Continuum set out overleaf.

The plan uses a range of repetitions from 6-15. The strength work is based on the amount of weight that you can lift for 6 repetitions. This Six Repetition Maximum is unique to you, your body type, sex, height, weight fitness level, general health, motivation and age. For each of the 6 repetitions, you must maintain correct body alignment, controlled, precise movements and a natural breathing rhythm. Your individual Six Repetition

---

CORRECT TECHNIQUE FOR STRENGTH WORK

- ✦ Move slowly, smoothly and with control as though moving underwater.
- ✦ Find a steady rhythm.
- ✦ Breath naturally throughout. Avoid holding your breath as this builds tension and can cause unnecessary increases in blood pressure.
- ✦ Maintain joint alignment throughout (see page 56).
- ✦ Check posture throughout. (Performing in front of a mirror works well.)
- ✦ Rest in between each set.
- ✦ When your muscles begin to ache, burn, or feel tired do one more repetition only and stop. Then rest or move a little to release tension and refresh the muscles.

STRENGTH CONTINUUM
No of Repetitions

| 6 | 10 | 12 | 15 |

Strength   Endurance

Maximum is something you can calculate by feel; always err on the side of caution, starting with a light weight and perfecting your technique and performance for some weeks before progressing to heavier weights.

Guidelines for successful, safe strength work

For successful, safe strength work follow the stages set out below:

STAGE 1

+ To learn the exercise technique, begin **without** a weight.
+ Progress to a light weight.
+ Only when you can do 12 to 15 repetitions with correct technique should you progress to resting for 2 minutes before repeating the set.
+ When your workout consists of two sets of 12 to 15 repetitions performed comfortably and correctly, progress to Stage 2.

STAGE 2

+ Increase the weight to one that you can lift for 6 to 8 repetitions. This is now your new six repetition maximum.
+ Start with one set of six repetitions of each exercise.
+ Keeping the weight the same, increase the number of sets until you can lift first two and then three sets of 6 to 8 repetitions.
+ Only when you can do this comfortably has the time come to move on to Stage 3 – increasing the weight to continue your strength improvements.

STAGE 3

+ Keep the number of sets and repetitions the same, but as the work becomes easy increase the amount of weight that you lift.

It is important to 'rest' in between each set either by stretching, or working a different muscle group or simply by being still. Alternating upper and lower body exercises also helps to provide a longer recovery time. Allow two minutes before working the same muscle again and at least a two day break before repeating strength work for a particular part of the body.

NB Remember it is better to do **one** set of each exercise than do two or three sets of just a few of them.

At the end of the session you should feel that you have worked hard without being exhausted, with muscles tired but not fatigued or sore. Put equal amounts of effort and control into both the lifting and lowering phases of each movement. Always finish with additional stretching and mobilising exercises to release any tension and to lengthen and refresh the muscles. If your muscles are sore and stiff the next day, even after stretching, you need to reduce the weight a little until your muscles are fitter.

HOW HARD, HOW LONG, HOW OFTEN?

To make sure you keep your new found muscular strength, do: two sessions a week *NOT* on consecutive days, each session comprising one to three sets of 6 to 8 repetitions at 6 to 7 on the Borg Scale
OR
For local muscular endurance do two sets of 12 to 15 repetitions of 8 to 10 major muscle groups and 5 to 7 on the Borg Scale.

This may seem daunting, but it's all taken care of in the Fitness For Life Plan. Once you have learned the techniques, the exercise order and found the correct weights for you to start with, you can do one set of strength work for 8 to 10 major muscle groups in under 12 minutes.

Stretching

The final type of muscle conditioning exercise is stretching for flexibility. We train flexibility by lengthening the muscles to increase the range of movement at the joints.

A unique feature of the Fitness For Life Plan is that there are stretches throughout the muscle conditioning to provide active 'rests' from the strength exercises and avoid the tension that may be felt when the stretches are done all together.

Careful, controlled stretching is a daily must. It can transform your posture, lengthen your spine, give you an ease of movement you may have thought had gone for ever. Tasks such as tying shoelaces, looking over your shoulder, will never be a problem if you follow The Fitness For Life Plan.

The flexibility training consists of both **maintenance** and **developmental** stretching. Maintenance stretching returns the muscles to their natural length and maintains them in good working order. Developmental stretching 'increases' the length of the muscles, and so improves their range of movement.

When the muscles are at their warmest, they are ready for the developmental stretches; these are held for longer, allowing time for you to move further into the stretch once the feeling of tension has eased. This movement needs to be done very gradually. The stretch positions need to be completely comfortable and thus may differ for each of us.

The stretching activities also begin the vital final '**cool down**' process that continues with relaxation and remobilisation exercises.

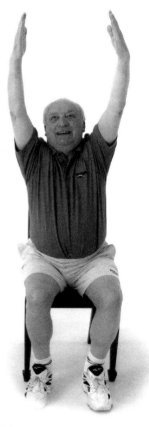

STRETCH!

HOW HARD, HOW LONG, HOW OFTEN?

For stretching, The Fitness for Life Plan recommends:

+ DAILY stretching.
+ 10 to 12 muscle groups three times (developmentally for any areas that are inflexible).
+ Maintenance stretches 8 to 10 seconds.
+ Developmental stretches up to 30 seconds.

The Borg Scale is not appropriate here, as it measures how hard we are working. In stretching, the feeling should be one of ease, of concentrated effort but no strain. Allow correct body alignment, the position, gravity and your muscles to do the work. Using the relaxation techniques that follow to release tension in both the muscle being stretched and the surrounding muscles, can make a great difference to your stretching progress and resulting suppleness.

Relaxation and remobilising

These complete the workout and cool down process. Relaxation relieves tension and stress and brings a renewed flow of energy. With practice it can help you to cope with stress so that you perform better in everyday life. Relaxation should not be confused with a state of lazy collapse, rather it is a state that allows your blood and energy to flow freely and your mind to function clearly. It makes you feel much more alive, gives you more control over your life. Relaxation has to be learned. 'Relax' is not an order that our bodies can understand or do at will.

The relaxation technique we recommend is based on the well respected and simple to follow Laura Mitchell Method of Physiological Relaxation. Working systematically round the body you follow an easy-to-remember action list to move specific body parts in a particular way, hold that position, then stop – and you will find that body part is relaxed.

The Laura Mitchell method of physiological relaxation

The instructions can be applied whether you are lying on your back or sitting in a high-backed chair, or against a wall. It is important to be warm and comfortable before you begin. You are going to:

✦ Give a series of definite 'action' orders that your body can follow e.g. pull the shoulders down; lift, stretch, push.

✦ Give yourself an order to **stop** doing the action.

✦ Feel the new positions and register them in your mind, focusing on the feeling in your **skin** and **joints**, not in your muscles.

Apply these three 'action orders' to each part of the body in turn, as listed below:

1 Pull your shoulders down away from your ears as far as you can.
2 Lift your elbows slightly outwards, away from your ribs and lower your hands to your thighs.
3 Stretch your fingers and thumbs long and wide.
4 Turn your hips and knees outwards.
5 Push your feet away from your head, slowly.
6 Push your body into the support (floor/chair)
7 Press your head and spine against the floor/chair. Hold for a second. Stop doing it. Feel and register the new position of ease.
8 Keep your breathing even and slow.
9 Make sure your teeth are apart, your tongue is in the lower part of your mouth and your lips moist.
10 Close your eyes.
11 Pucker your forehead into a frown then mentally smooth your forehead from your eyebrows to your hairline, over the top of your head and down the back of your neck.
12 Repeat the whole sequence a little more quickly.

Enjoy your newly relaxed body for a few moments, then stretch your limbs before getting up.

Practising the technique for even a minute or two at the end of your workout can bring a feeling of being deeply relaxed and rested, as well as refreshed. It can be done any time, anywhere to calm nerves, renew energy or ease niggling tension.

After lying or sitting still for any length of

time it is very important to get moving again **slowly**. Leaping up can cause dizziness, cramps and numb limbs. It is best to sit comfortably for two or three minutes, performing some of the joint mobilising exercises from the warm up, and repeating one or two of the seated stretches, before standing up. These low level body warming moves will 'revitalise' your body and get you ready to swing back into your day.

LEARN TO RECOGNISE THE SIGNS OF STRESS

Most of us know *how* it feels! Here are some practical warning signs to help you catch it early:
+ Head and body bent forward, chin jutting down or outwards.
+ Jaw clamped, teeth clenched.
+ Shoulders up and tight.
+ Elbows bent up and arms hugging the chest.
+ Fingers clenched.
+ Legs crossed; foot tapping.
+ Breathing held or quickened.

The exercise-essentials session

The next chapter will initiate you into the essentials of exercise, with the tips and tricks that fitness, sports and exercise professionals use to get the most out of their training programmes. As with everything, a few quality moves will produce the results you want much more quickly than many badly performed exercises. So take time to study the instructions and master the 'exercise essentials' before you begin, then give each exercise your very best effort. This will guarantee a truly remarkable and lasting return. Your body deserves the very best care you can give it.

The Fitness For Life Plan also shows how, without actually 'exercising', you can make your life a mini workout. Such everyday actions as getting in and out of a chair, up and down from the floor, walking to the shops, gardening, standing at the bus stop, done correctly, strengthen and protect our bodies, helping to prevent illness and falls and making all the difference to our enjoyment of life (see Chapter 7)

CHAPTER 5

The exercise essentials

Before we begin to exercise there are a few more essentials that we would recommend you master, because they form the basis of all safe and effective exercise and are used constantly throughout the Fitness For Life Plan.

Posture

Good posture is essential if you are going to reap the full benefit from exercising. It is also one of the secrets of ageless ageing. It gives a look and feeling of energy, vitality and ease that makes the years drop away.

Good posture is when all the parts of the body are correctly aligned and therefore the minimum amount of stress and strain is placed on the body and its joints. Good posture is relaxed, needs less energy and muscle activity to maintain it; the body looks balanced and efficient; movement is smooth,

easy and economical. (Poor posture creates unequal tension in the body, so that movements tend to be jerky, clumsy and look uncomfortable.)

Habitual misuse

The secret of good posture is to put every part of the body exactly where it is designed to be. It sounds easy and should come naturally, so why is it so hard to achieve? The answer is that our posture has developed over the years in direct response to the pull of gravity, our frame of mind and the habits of a lifetime. The actions and tasks of our daily lives overwork some tissues and underwork others, leading to a change in the body's natural shape.

Sitting at a desk, bent over for hours at a time, can lead to a weakening and over-stretching of the muscles across the back, a permanent rounding of the shoulders and curvature of the spine. Carrying a heavy bag on the same side each day, sitting for long periods watching TV or driving can cause hip and thigh muscles to tighten and shorten, and the pelvis to tip. All this may be accompanied by a sagging chest and weak tummy muscles which together can cause the spine to develop an exaggerated arch or curve, creating strain in the lower back. These two postural problems alone cause hundreds of thousands of lost working days, great discomfort, and pain. In the long term, because joints are pulled out of alignment, they can lead to the development of *osteoarthritis* and severe disability. Even badly fitting footwear or high heels can cause damaging structural changes throughout the body. Fortunately, you can prevent a lot of these problems with postural training.

Poor posture is the repeated use of lazy unco-ordinated patterns that finally become habits. Habits can be changed. With a bit of effort you can learn good posture. Then, the skeleton works well. It carries your weight with minimum strain, enabling you to perform a wide range of complex movements and to enjoy the benefits of a free flow of blood and energy around the body. Good posture relies on correct spinal alignment. The head should balance freely at the top of the spine. The shoulders should be directly over the hips so that the weight of the head and trunk are transmitted evenly through the curves of the spine to the large bony basin of the pelvis and out to the legs. This ensures a full, natural range of movement at every joint, balance and stability. It also minimises joint wear and tear, and muscle fatigue.

Both strength and flexibility in the main postural muscles are essential for maintaining this correct alignment. Strong back, shoulders, buttock, thighs and abdominal muscles, and pliable muscles at the front of the chest and the thighs are all important for resisting gravity and maintaining good posture.

The Active Living approach to posture

Much of our daily lives involves being in one position, or carrying out often repeated small actions. Unless we counteract the ill effects by taking exercise, correcting our position wherever we can, and getting up and moving about at regular intervals, occupational posture faults will inevitably develop. Good posture will help prevent much of the wear and tear and loss of height that tends to be associated with old age. A recent survey showed that active older people are considerably taller than their non active counterparts; they have escaped some of the shrinking! The difference in our general appearance will also be remarkable; good posture makes us look and feel years younger.

Each day:
✦ Check your posture constantly.
✦ Get up every 30 minutes or so. Never sit for too long.
✦ Change sides when carrying heavy shopping.
✦ Wear shoulder bags on different sides.
✦ Be conscious of lengthening your body upwards and forwards as you stand up.
✦ Note which leg you lead to stand up with, and then use the other leg to lead for two weeks. Then try to alternate regularly.

This routine may feel strange at first but each daily action will help to improve strength, balance, co-ordination and control of movement.

Posture Check

POOR POSTURE

- ✦ Neck and head drooping downwards and forwards.
- ✦ Chin jutting forwards.
- ✦ Eyes dropped, shoulders rounded and stooped.
- ✦ Rib cage collapsed into the hips.
- ✦ Shoulders up.
- ✦ Back rounded, chest sunken inwards, restricting air flow.
- ✦ Pelvis tilted incorrectly.
- ✦ Back rounded and shortened and abdominals slack.
- ✦ Weight unevenly distributed and mainly on heels.
- ✦ Knees sagging over the toes and rolling inwards.
- ✦ Plumb line wanders all over the place = uneven stress on joints and muscles.

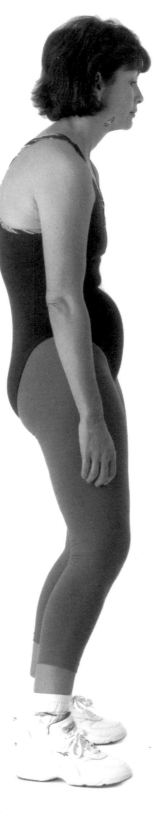

GOOD POSTURE

- ✦ The neck and head lengthened upwards.
- ✦ Chin parallel to the floor.
- ✦ Eyes looking straight ahead.
- ✦ Shoulders down and away from the ears.
- ✦ Ribs lifted up away from the hips.
- ✦ Breathing easy and regular.
- ✦ Pelvis correctly tilted to allow natural curves in the back.
- ✦ Lower back lengthened and abdominals tightened.
- ✦ Weight placed evenly over both feet.
- ✦ Knees soft (relaxed) and over the ankles.
- ✦ Plumb line is straight from crown to floor = minimum stress.

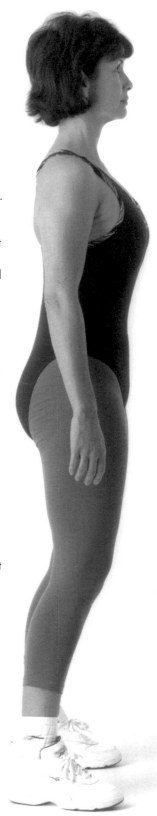

The exercise approach to posture

The Fitness For Life Plan focuses attention on all the postural muscles. The Warm Up and Muscle Conditioning with Flexibility Stretching Sections offer comprehensive postural training. They lengthen the muscles that gravity, life and bad habits have shortened, and strengthen the muscles that help to keep the body erect. Let's look at an example of good and bad habits and then you can assess your posture so that you know exactly what you need to work on.

Your posture assessment

A simple way to assess your posture is to imagine tracing a line through the body that passes from a point between your ankles to a point at the centre of the crown of your head.

From the back Your ankles, knee creases, buttock creases, shoulder blades, shoulder lines and ears should be exactly level when measured horizontally across the line.

From the side The line should pass just in front of your outer ankle bone and in front of the middle of the knee, through the hip, lower spine, middle of the shoulder, upper spine, the ear and out through the centre of the crown.

From the front The plumb line should divide your body into two. Your head is held

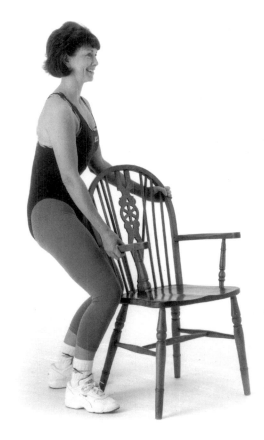

The correct posture for lifting is described on page 138

erect, tilted neither left nor right, and each shoulder and hip bone is level with its partner. When your arms are held out in front at shoulder level, the palms are the same height from the floor. Your shin bones are fairly straight, not bow legged, kneecaps the same height and facing forwards, knees over ankles, feet turned slightly outwards with your weight resting on the mid line of each foot.

The real challenge comes when you begin to move. Good posture applies both in stillness (**static posture**) and in movement (**dynamic posture**). And there's no better time to practise than when exercising. Performing exercise from a sound foundation will help to keep it safe and more effective too.

POSTURE SHORTHAND

This **Three Point Check** can be done whenever you have a spare moment; at the bus stop, waiting for the kettle to boil, watching television, at a party, going for a walk. And of course, throughout your exercise sessions.
1) **Lengthen** the neck up as you
2) **Ease** the shoulders down and
3) **Lengthen** the base of your spine towards the floor.

Checklist of anti-tension adjustments

Run through these small but significant anti-tension, anti-ageing adjustments from top to toe both when exercising and throughout your day.

✦ Eyes soft, not staring.

✦ Are you holding your breath? Breathe out easily.

✦ Lips soft and lightly closed, not pursed or open.

✦ Tongue at ease in your mouth, not clamped tightly to the roof of the mouth.

✦ Teeth slightly apart, not clamped together.

✦ Stand tall, don't sag in the middle.

✦ Lengthen your spine upwards and do not arch your back however slightly, knees and elbows 'soft' (relaxed).

✦ Toes alive!

✦ Do the **Three Point Check** (see page 54) whenever you remember.

The posture check has instant results – just by correcting your posture, you will be taller, trimmer and feel stronger and more positive.

Care of the joints during exercise

This is vital and individual. We all have the same types of joint but there is a big variation between individuals in the way our joints behave – our range of movement, joint stability and flexibility. Genetic factors such as body type and size, physical training, inactivity, disease and injury can all affect the structure and function of our joints.

There are certain safety guidelines that can be applied to all joint actions. It is up to each of us to make the small adjustments that ensure our range of movement feels comfortable. This improves as our fitness improves. As we get older allowing time for this adjustment to activity is important, knees in particular can be troublesome to begin with and then 'free up' as the body adapts.

Careless alignment and unsafe moves can result in damage to the cartilage, ligaments, joint capsules and muscles; but complete inactivity can have a similar effect. Loss of mobility, joint stiffness and tight or sagging muscles are major contributors to balance and reflex problems and disability as we grow older.

On the other hand, correct technique and moves that respect the range of actions the joint is designed to do, can result in a healthier cartilage, more pliable, stable ligaments and a well preserved joint capsule and movement range. It is not only **what** you do but the **way** that you do it that will make the difference.

Care of the back

Spinal alignment is the key. The position of the pelvis and the strength of the abdominals is crucial to support the back in sitting, standing, lying and all trunk movement. The Pelvic Tilt is the most effective way of achieving this (see page 55)

Care of the knees

The knee joint is one of the most vulnerable in the body. It has to be strong enough to bear your whole body weight in actions such as walking and stair climbing and yet it has to have enough 'give' to let you get up and down from chairs, the floor etcetera. The structure of the knee joint is that of a hinge; it allows movement in one plane only. It can bend (flex) or straighten (extend). Tight ligaments help to form a strong joint and, contrary to popular belief, the knee is not built to rotate or move sideways. If it does, injury can occur.

The pelvic tilt

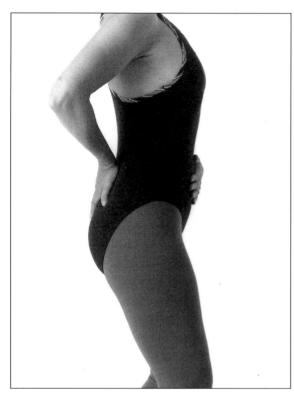

Incorrect tilt

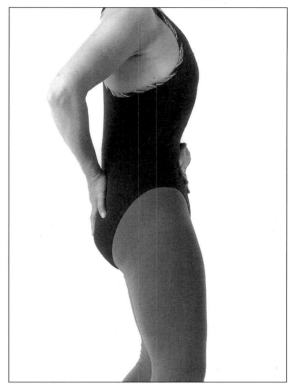

Correct tilt

PREPARATION

Place one hand on your tummy and the other on your lower back. Allow your back to hollow a little. Feel the pelvis tilt **incorrectly** and the tummy pushing outwards.

ACTION

Tilt your pelvis the opposite way bringing your hip bones up towards your face. Feel your bottom move under and your back lengthen. Notice the hollow almost disappear and feel your tummy moving away from the front hand. Rest.

Slide your hands away, placing them by your sides. Repeat the pelvic tilt, breathing out as you pull the tummy muscles in tight. Try to pull your navel through to your backbone. Feel your tummy become firm. Breathe in

and release gently. Rest and repeat. Keep the ribs lifted away from your hips throughout, especially if seated.

✦ Keep the back of your neck lengthened.
✦ Avoid hollowing your back as you release.
✦ Avoid flattening your back completely as you tilt.
✦ Try to maintain the pelvic tilt with tight abdominals. Once you've mastered this in one position, practise it standing and, if possible, when walking, climbing stairs, lying on one side, going from standing to sitting to lying until you feel really confident. You will be using it again and again in the exercises featured in Chapter 6.

One of the muscles that controls the knee is attached to the ligaments and cartilage. This gives a bit more ease of movement but also makes the joint more vulnerable to injury.

Knee bends form the basis for many of the exercises in the Fitness For Life Plan, and for many actions in everyday life. If you are not used to regular exercise, or if you already have some difficulties with your knees, it is especially important to start gradually with good technique and keep knee bends shallow, until your muscles strengthen sufficiently to control the joint.

Knee problems often occur as the result of:

1 Weak thigh muscles A gentle approach can help not only to prevent injury but to promote well balanced leg strength and a more age-resistant joint.

2 Unsafe exercises The knee becomes extremely vulnerable as soon as the degree of bend is greater than 90 degrees (when the bottom is below the level of the knees). This places considerable strain on the ligaments which, once overstretched, can no longer stabilise the joint so securely.

3 Poor alignment Alignment is another key knee safety factor. The knees should always be directly in line with the hips and the ankles. In the bent position the knees should be over the front of the foot and you should always be able to see the big toe on the inside of your knee.

4 Poor performance Another movement that requires care and skill, is straightening your knee from the bent position. Take care not to snap, or 'lock', the knee joint straight,

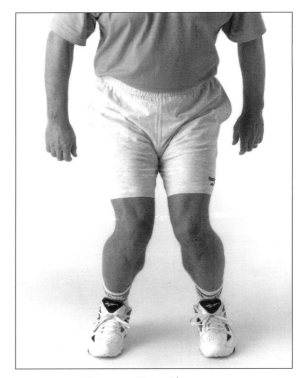

Incorrect Knee Alignment

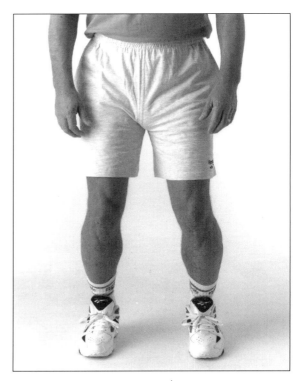

Correct Knee Alignment

because this jars the joint structures and increases joint wear and tear. Controlling the straightening action until the joint is extended, 'soft' but not 'locked', can help to stabilise the knee. Although this is most important during weight-bearing exercise, it is also relevant for seated muscular conditioning and multi gym work.

Care of the elbows and shoulders

The elbows, like the knees, are hinge joints and though weight bearing is less of an issue, they share many of the same safety points. 'Locking out' tends to be even more common because the elbow joint is less stable. Movements using the arm in the straight position are rare in life and we are relatively unskilled at performing them. Ensure there is always a slight bend or 'softness' in the elbow even in the straight position. This is crucial when working with equipment as 'locking out' can lead to hyper-extension and injury. To ensure correct alignment in weight bearing such as in the box position below, your hands should always face forward, with your wrists under your shoulders and elbows bent directly in line with your shoulder joints.

The shoulders, like the hips, are ball and socket joints and capable of a big range of movement. The shoulder is particularly mobile and, again, is stabilised only by the ligaments and muscles. It is essential when performing all arm movements to avoid flinging actions that may take the shoulder beyond its comfortable range and cause unnecessary shoulder injuries.

Preparation position for box press-up

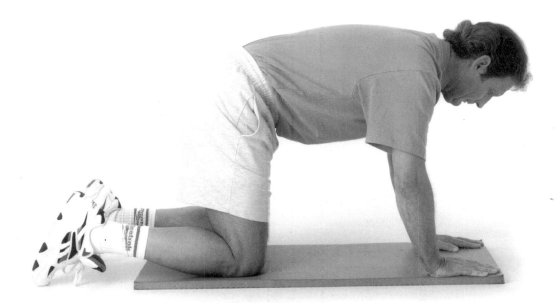

Correct spinal alignment in abdominal exerise

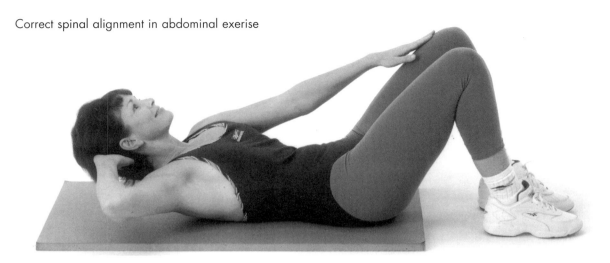

Care of the neck

When performing the abdominal lifts, the upper spine should be kept long (i.e. not curled in) as this places unnecessary strain on the vertebrae of the neck and upper back. This is particularly important in post menopausal women or anyone who has *osteoporosis.*

People often experience great tension in the neck when doing abdominal work, because they are 'leading' with the neck and/or not tightening the abdominals sufficiently first. Always try to keep the neck 'free'. Resting the head in one hand as you lift can work well. Otherwise return to basic abdominal contractions with the pelvic tilt until your muscles are stronger (see page 55).

Care of the ankles, knees and feet

'Springing', skipping, jumping and stepping actions increase strength and power, bone density, balance and reflexes. However, any of these actions require correct take off and landing techniques to safely absorb the impact.

To reduce impact to a minimum, bend at the ankles, knees and hips, and work through the feet, both before and after the springing action. This will achieve maximum lift on the take off and maximum cushioning on the landing. Keeping your body tall and aligned throughout helps the natural spinal curves, the back and the leg muscles to absorb the shock of the landing.

Jumping or 'springing' technique

✦ Prepare by bending your knees and ankles. Keeping your knees directly over your toes, push up through your thighs and feet, lifting the body upwards onto your toes and into the air.

✦ Keep your body lengthened upwards and point your toes downwards.

✦ Land through your feet, toes, ball, heel, bending your knees and ankles again to spread the load.

✦ Control the landing movement by tightening your thigh muscles, bending a little deeper and keeping your heels on the floor until your weight is evenly centred over both feet.

✦ Spring again or return to an upright position.

NOTE: Never jump without a full warm-up.

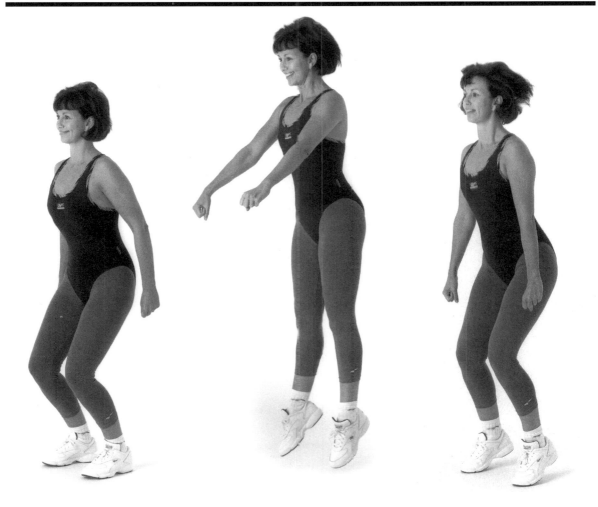

Jumping – preparation   In the air   Landing

There are 4 jumping patterns:
+ 2 feet to 2 feet
+ 2 feet to 1 foot
+ 1 foot to 1 foot
+ 1 foot to 2 feet

The safest, most effective, is the two feet to two feet jump. To prevent any possibility of a fall, it is a good idea to start practising the jumps holding on to a chair. If you have a joint condition that would make jumping inappropriate, are new to exercise, or simply don't enjoy it, just do the first stage of lifting on to your toes. Do it with all the energy of a jump without the actual take off and it can be just as much fun.

Prevention of falls

Some actions used in general exercise sessions, although fun, can be risky and are best omitted. The cross over step or 'grapevine' is a good example. The action stresses the knee and lower back considerably. The real danger though, is catching your back foot on the heel of the foot in front. Even if the first few repetitions are done skilfully, tiredness can lead to carelessness. The Fitness For Life Plan uses only safe options such as simple side stepping which can be just as enjoyable and can work the body twice as hard because you are more secure.

Vital anytime, anywhere exercises

Below are some simple exercises for your hands and feet that can be done any time and anywhere – watching television, sitting in the garden, etc. There is also a pelvic floor exercise which ideally should be done every day; fit it into your daily routine so that it becomes as automatic as brushing your teeth.

Finger mobilisers

PURPOSE

To keep the small joints of the hand mobile, to improve the nimbleness and co-ordination of fingers and thumbs.

PREPARATION

Stand or sit tall with good posture.

ACTION

Position your legs, knees and feet hip-width apart, and rest your palms on your thighs. Bending comfortably at the elbow, lift your forearms up towards your shoulders with fingers spread wide. Soften the fingers slightly to allow ease of movement. Make large, slow circles with each finger in turn. End by spreading your fingers wide again. Then, making sure the fingers don't bang against each other, shake out your fingers to release any tension.

REST AND REPEAT SEVERAL TIMES.

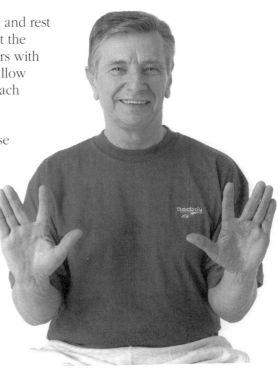

ALTERNATIVE

Spread your fingers wide as before and bring your thumb across your palm to touch the tip of the little finger, making a large, round O shape. Return to the spread position. Repeat the move with each finger in turn. Rest and repeat. If you have difficulty doing this exercise, work one hand at a time and use the free hand to gently assist the fingers of the other hand.

Wrist mobilisers

PURPOSE

To keep the wrists mobile and to improve co-ordination.

PREPARATION

Stand or sit tall as before.

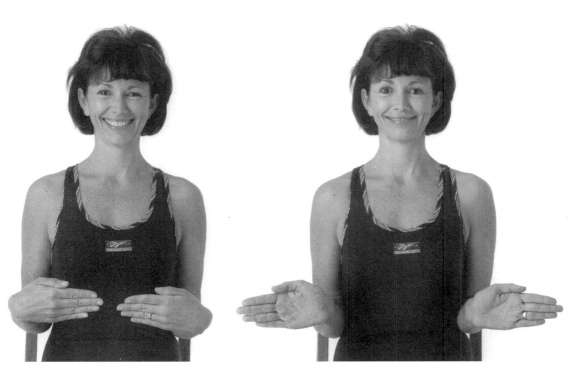

ACTION

Position your arms by your sides and bend the elbows so that your forearms are held out in front, at right angles to your upper arms, with the palms facing each other.

Bend at the wrist to form another right angle, taking your hand and finger tips inwards as far as possible. Hold for a moment. Reverse the movement, taking your hand and fingers outwards as far as possible. Rest and repeat several times, ending with the fingers inwards. Try to keep your elbows pressed into your sides and your forearms still throughout.

ALTERNATIVE

Keeping the arms still as before, move your hands in circles from the wrists, up, in, down and out. After making several inward circles, rest, then repeat with outward circles. Rest. Finally, release any tension by 'playing a piano' with your fingers and thumbs.

Vital anytime, anywhere exercises

Wrist strengtheners

PURPOSE

To strengthen the wrist bones and muscles, to prevent fractures and improve grip strength

PREPARATION

Standing or sitting tall, as before.

ACTION

As for wrist mobilisers, arms by your sides and bent at the elbows, palms up, holding a tennis ball in each hand. Squeeze the balls for a count of 6. Rest and repeat x 10. Keep breathing naturally throughout.

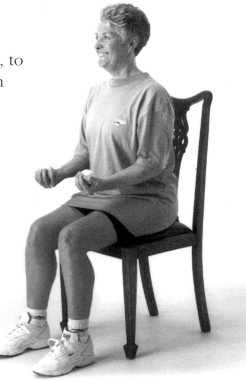

Ankle circles

PURPOSE

To keep the ankles free from stiffness and to improve circulation.

PREPARATION

Stand or sit tall as before. Your weight supported on a wall, chair, or, as shown, between two chairs.

ACTION

Transfer your weight to one leg, and slowly circle your foot and ankle one way and then the other. Try to keep your knee and shin still. Rest and repeat several times. Then transfer your weight to the other leg and repeat.

This is not a balance exercise, so if standing, use a support and take care to keep the opposite knee slightly bent to support the weight more comfortably. Imagine you have a pencil at the end of your big toe. Make large, slow, smooth circles.

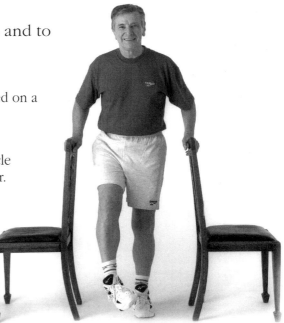

Pelvic floor strengtheners

These are most important for maintaining function and control of the pelvic floor in both men and women. Loss of bladder control can cause great unhappiness and distress but much can be achieved by doing these simple exercises every day.

PURPOSE

To strengthen the muscles of the bladder opening and the back passage (pelvic floor).

PREPARATION

Sit, stand, or lie down on your side with knees bent up, or kneel; whichever position you choose, gravity helps you to feel the muscles. Position your legs slightly apart. Check your posture and breathe out, to consciously release any tension.

ACTION

Try to draw up and close the back passage and 'the waterworks' or urinary passage, as if to stop yourself from urinating. Tighten the muscles even more, deep inside. Hold for a count of 6. Then let go slowly. Repeat 6 times. Repeat whole sequence 6 times per day, taking care not to hold the breath – breathe evenly and naturally.

In addition, to work the quick muscle fibres, repeat the action as fast as possible. Hold for one second and release. Repeat once a day. Breathe evenly and naturally.

NOTE Nothing should move on the outside! All the action is on the inside. So avoid tightening your abdominals or buttock muscles.

If you find it difficult to feel the muscles, try tightening 'the waterworks' first. If this doesn't work, try stopping the actual flow of urine in mid stream a few times, just to find the spot. This is also a good way to test you are doing the exercises correctly. Do not do this mid-stream test regularly, as back flow could cause infection.

We are now fully versed in the Exercise Essentials and ready to begin. This is the moment we have been waiting for. The Fitness for Life Exercise Plan. *Let's go!*

CHAPTER 6

The Fitness for Life Exercise Plan

This exercise plan is designed to help you keep active, defy the years, and fight the real enemy – inactivity. You will soon find yourself looking better, feeling full of vitality, having more energy and strength for every day tasks, and a better quality of life. THE PLAN provides a safe, effective, comprehensive and progressive system of exercise for the health and fitness of the whole body. A system that conditions and strengthens, stretches and lengthens, energises and refreshes, relaxes and destresses; that offers alternatives and enough variety to suit everyone. It targets bones and posture, balance and power, stamina, speed and strength; flexibility and mobility, co-ordination and control. It trains these and other fitness factors to counter the health problems that were once thought to be the inevitable, irreversible process of ageing. Today we know them to be

largely the result of inactivity and loss of fitness.

There is increasing evidence that regular moderate exercise helps prevent conditions such as osteoporosis, late onset diabetes, hypertension, heart disease and stroke, incontinence, bowel problems, leg swelling and skin ulceration.

At every age regular exercise is known to balance blood pressure and cholesterol, help weight control, reduce tiredness and postural problems, improve sleep, skin, hair, nails and bones, and all the body tissues, as well as boost the immune system, confidence and energy.

Each workout should leave you feeling more alive and positive, more relaxed and able to cope with, and really enjoy, life. Bending and stretching will become easier, you'll be stronger, more agile, less breathless, more energetic. You will develop an awareness of your own body and posture, and be able to correct it at will. You will take a pride in your movement skills and performance, and a pleasure in the feeling that fitness gives.

Please note that we have used mirror images for the photographs in the exercise section. This is to make the exercises easier to follow; refer to the photographs as if you were watching the teacher in a class.

The Fitness For Life Plan options

It is time to consider the options that the Fitness For Life Plan provides.

The Plan is arranged in four separate sections: The Warm Up, the Stamina Conditioning Section, the Muscle Conditioning, Strength and Stretch Section and the Relaxation and Remobilising section. Each is of vital importance to all-round fitness. Each focuses on different components of fitness and is designed to ensure maximum safety and benefit.

The table on the right arranges these sections into five clear combinations, to give plenty of choice and flexibility. On days when you have to miss a lengthier workout, the Daily Dozen (selected highlights of the complete workout – see page 67), which takes 20 minutes, is ideal. And if you have only 10 minutes to spare, the warm-up alone is a good way to start or end the day. For very little effort, you get great returns. Just getting the circulation going will stimulate your body and brain, and bring that general feeling of vitality that makes life so much more enjoyable, and sleep come more easily.

The options range from the short and 'easy does it', to longer and more challenging. If you are just beginning, start gently with Workout 1 and progress slowly and steadily. For the fitter exerciser Workouts 4 and 5 are ideal.

Workout options

Workout 1, The Warm Up
This workout simply involves the Warm Up (pages 68–91) and takes about 10 minutes. It can be lengthened by repetition.   10 mins +

Workout 2, Mini Conditioning
This involves the Warm Up (pages 68–91), the Daily Dozen (page 99) and Muscle Fitness exercises (see page 110).   15 mins

Workout 3, Muscle Conditioning
This involves the Warm Up (pages 68–91) followed by the Muscle Conditioning Plan (strengthening and local endurance exercises and flexibility stretches, pages 102–134) and ends with Remobilisers (page 135)   30 mins

Workout 4, Stamina Conditioning
This involves the Warm Up (pages 68–91) followed by the Stamina (Aerobic) Conditioning Plan (pages 93–101), then all of the stretches in the Muscle Conditioning Plan (beginning on page 118) and ends with Remobilisers (page 135)   35 mins

Workout 5, Complete Conditioning
This workout for the fitter exerciser involves the Warm Up (pages 68–91) followed by the Stamina (Aerobic) Conditioning Plan (pages 93–101), and the Muscle Conditioning Plan strengthening and endurance exercises with flexibility stretches (pages 102–134), the Relaxation (page 132) and finishes with the Remobilisers (page 135)   50 mins

Fitness For Life Week

Once you've got into the swing of things you may want to plan ahead, decide which to do on different days and write it down. Your Fitness for Life Week might then look like this. Remember, your main aim is to progress at the right pace for you – don't push yourself too hard. This suggested week's activity may be some way ahead; but you *will* achieve it sooner or later.

Sunday	10 mins: Warm Up + a restful (or energetic!) non-workout day
Monday	50 mins: Warm Up + 1 full workout
Tuesday	30 mins: Warm Up + 1 muscle conditioning workout
Wednesday	35 mins: Warm Up + 1 stamina (aerobic) workout **or** brisk activity of your choice + flexibility stretches
Thursday	50 mins: Warm Up + 1 full workout
Friday	30 mins: Warm Up + 1 brisk activity of your choice + flexibility stretches
Saturday	35 mins: Warm Up + 1 muscle conditioning workout

Exercising – safety guidelines

✦ Allow 2 hours after eating and 1 hour after drinking tea or coffee.

✦ Drink water (not tea or coffee) before, during and after exercise.

✦ Wear appropriate footwear and comfortable cotton clothing.

✦ Make sure the room is warm and well ventilated.

✦ Listen to your body. Never work with pain – stop immediately.

✦ Never work to the point of exhaustion.

✦ Know the difference between discomfort, pain and fatigue.

✦ Always work at your own level and progress slowly.

✦ Always warm up and cool down for 5 minutes.

✦ Avoid being over ambitious at the beginning if you are unfit.

✦ Take a pride in correct technique. Always move rhythmically and with control.

✦ Keep your breathing regular throughout.

Memory joggers

◆ Completely clear a space before you start and have any equipment handy.

◆ Make sure you have mastered the **exercise essentials**, including PELVIC TILT (Chapter 5) before you start.

◆ Check your **posture** before and during each exercise.

◆ **Repetitions** are the number of times to do the exercise.

◆ A **set** is a series of repetitions.

◆ Every exercise has **Technique Tips** to help you get the best results safely.

◆ Many exercises have a **seated alternative** and suggestions for **variety** and **progress**.

◆ **Always begin with the Warm Up** and always cool down with Flexibility Stretches and Remobilisation.

◆ No matter which workout combination you choose, try to fit all exercises marked **NB DAILY DOZEN** into your programme. For simplification, these 12 essential exercises are listed below.

Daily Dozen checklist

<table>
<tr><td></td><td></td><td>Page</td></tr>
<tr><td>1. **Posture Check**</td><td>To lengthen and realign body. An instant beauty treatment.</td><td>68</td></tr>
<tr><td>2. **Easy Walking**</td><td>To increase circulation – even better if it's done outdoors.</td><td>69</td></tr>
<tr><td>3. **Shoulder Circles**</td><td>To lubricate and increase mobility in the spine.</td><td>71</td></tr>
<tr><td>4. **Side Bends**</td><td>To lubricate and increase mobility in the spine.</td><td>72</td></tr>
<tr><td>5. **Trunk Twists**</td><td>To lubricate and increase rotational mobility in the spine.</td><td>73</td></tr>
<tr><td>6. **Ankle Activators**</td><td>To lubricate and increase mobility in the ankles.</td><td>78</td></tr>
<tr><td>7. **Inner Thigh Stretch**</td><td>To improve range of movement in the legs.</td><td>82</td></tr>
<tr><td>8. **Upward Side Stretch**</td><td>To maintain height.</td><td>88</td></tr>
<tr><td>9. **Chest Stretch**</td><td>To open the chest to improve breathing capacity.</td><td>89</td></tr>
<tr><td>10. **Back-of-Thigh Stretch**</td><td>To improve range of movement and reduce risks of injury in the legs.</td><td>90</td></tr>
<tr><td>11. **Thigh Strengthener**</td><td>To increase leg strength and power.</td><td>110</td></tr>
<tr><td>12. **Back Strengthener**</td><td>To strengthen the bones of the spine and improve posture.</td><td>114</td></tr>
</table>

Warm-up

WARM-UP: 10 MINUTES +

The **BODY WARMING EXERCISES** can be done every day. They begin the workout and will leave you feeling warmer, looser, more alive and ready for action. Although they have a swinging quality, keep the moves small and low at first, then, after you have loosened the joints with some mobility work, return to body warming and build the moves in size until you are involving the whole body. Feel the tension easing out of your muscles. Your breathing should be even and regular and only a little deeper than usual.

The **MOBILISING EXERCISES** are most effective if you isolate each movement, smoothly and gradually exploring the full range of movement at each joint, until you reach its largest possible movement. Feel the stiffness and twinges easing out of your joints, giving a looser, more mobile body.

The **STRETCHES** will lengthen out your muscles making you feel taller, more at ease and more aware of your body. Take time to get the alignment right and hold very still to effect the stretch safely. Keep warm-up stretching mild and light.

Every workout begins with a posture check (see right and page 52). Now you are ready for action!

GOOD POSTURE

+ The neck and head lengthened upwards.
+ Chin parallel to the floor.
+ Eyes looking straight ahead.
+ Shoulders down and away from the ears.
+ Ribs lifted up away from the hips.
+ Breast bone 'soft' and breathing easy and regular.
+ Pelvis correctly tilted to allow natural curves in the back.
+ Lower back lengthened and abdominals tightened.
+ Weight placed evenly over both feet.
+ Knees soft (not locked) and over the ankles.
+ Plumb line is straight from floor to crown = minimum stress.

N.B. DAILY DOZEN *no* **1**

WARM-UP EXERCISES

Easy walking

PURPOSE

To warm the muscles and promote the circulation

PREPARATION

✦ Stand tall with good posture, your feet about 3 inches apart and toes facing forward; your weight slightly more forward and upward than usual, and distributed evenly between both feet. Arms by your sides.

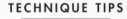

Easy walk 1 (on the spot)

ACTION

✦ Lift one heel and as you return it to the floor, lift the other heel up. Gradually increase the size of the movement by pushing up through the balls of the feet as you take the weight evenly from one foot to the other in an on-the-spot-foot-pedalling action.

CONTINUE FOR 30 SECONDS.

Easy walk 2 (travelling)

✦ Progress to travelling with this easy walking action round the room. Keep the strides fairly small and build to a strolling, enjoyable rhythm. Keep your arms low and move them naturally, in the opposite direction to your legs.

CONTINUE FOR 30 SECONDS THEN REPEAT EASY WALK 1 AND 2 ONCE MORE.

SEATED ALTERNATIVE

✦ Sit tall with good posture in an upright chair without arms to it. Hold the seat for support on Easy Walk 1. For Easy Walk 2 action, continue Easy Walk 1 in the legs and swing the arms as if marching.

NB If standing is possible with the support of a chair or wall, take this option as it will help to strengthen your bones.

> **TECHNIQUE TIPS**
>
> Roll your weight from the heel to the ball of your foot each time.
>
> ✦
>
> Keep the abdominals firm.
>
> ✦
>
> Keep your breathing regular and natural.

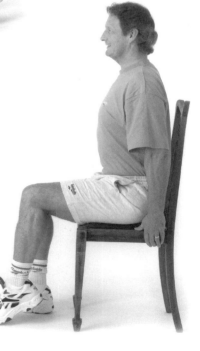

N.B. DAILY DOZEN *no* **2**

Shoulder mobilisers

PURPOSE

To loosen and lubricate shoulder joints,
maintain a good range of movement,
release tension and prevent rounded
shoulders. Both these exercises feel
very good to do.

PREPARATION

◆ Stand or sit tall with good
posture, your legs, knees and
feet hip width apart and your
arms resting lightly by your
sides.

Shoulder lift

ACTION

◆ Lift both shoulders up. Then,
taking care not to arch your
back, draw them down away
from your ears as far as you
can, at the same time
lengthening your neck.

**REPEAT 4 TIMES. REST AND
REPEAT.**

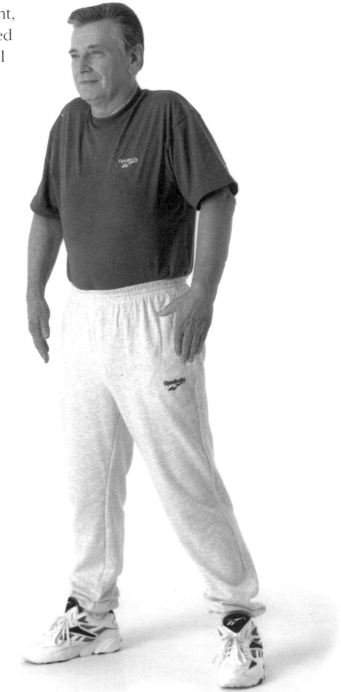

TECHNIQUE TIPS

Emphasise the backward
and downward movement.

◆

Feel the movement in your
shoulders and neck muscles.

◆

Keep your breathing regular
and the movement slow
and smooth.

Shoulder circles

ACTION

◆ Ease both shoulders forwards, upwards, backwards and down, taking care not to arch your back. Now move through each direction in a continuous circle, making this as large as possible. Hold the back and down position for a moment before releasing to start again.

REPEAT 4 TIMES. REST AND REPEAT.

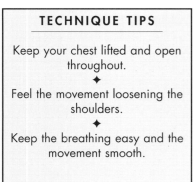

TECHNIQUE TIPS

Keep your chest lifted and open throughout.

◆

Feel the movement loosening the shoulders.

◆

Keep the breathing easy and the movement smooth.

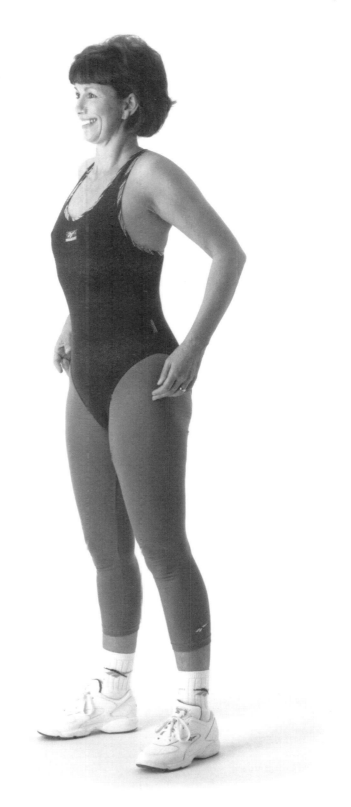

N.B. DAILY DOZEN no 3

Side bends

PURPOSE

To mobilise the spine, and improve body awareness and control of trunk moves.

PREPARATION

◆ Stand tall with good posture, your legs and feet shoulder width apart, your knees bent over your feet and your toes pointing naturally outwards. Your arms straight down by your sides. Do an extra pelvic tilt and pull in your abdominals to support your lower back.

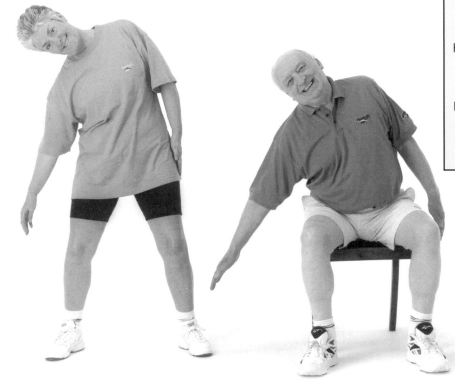

TECHNIQUE TIPS

Keep your weight even over both feet, your knees bent evenly.

◆

Keep breathing easily and move with control.

◆

Keep the weight even over both hips and avoid lifting off the seat.

ACTION

◆ Keeping the pelvic tilt steady and knees bent, bend slowly to one side, sliding your hand down parallel with your leg, taking your ear towards your shoulder while keeping your neck and back in a straight line. Avoid arching your back or leaning backwards or forwards. Keep the ribs lifted away from the waist.

◆ Return to the start; check your posture and repeat the exercise to the other side.

REPEAT 4 TIMES.

SEATED ALTERNATIVE

◆ Sit tall with good posture, your legs and feet shoulder width apart, your knees directly over your ankles and your feet facing forwards. Your arms straight down beside your hips.

◆ Keeping a firm pelvic tilt and the ribs lifted, slide your arm down in line with your hip. Avoid leaning forwards or backwards. Return to the start, check your posture and repeat the exercise to the other side.

REPEAT 4 TIMES.

N.B. DAILY DOZEN no 4

Trunk twists

PURPOSE

To mobilise the middle and upper parts of the spine, in order to maintain good upper body movement.

PREPARATION

✦ Stand tall with good posture, your legs and feet hip width apart, your knees bent and over your toes, your arms at chest level, bent at the elbows, with forearms resting on one another.

ACTION

✦ Keeping your hips and knees facing forwards, and your knees over the toes, lengthen your body upwards and slowly turn your head, shoulders and arms round to one side as far as you can. Keep your shoulders down throughout. Return to the start position and repeat to other side.

REPEAT 4 TIMES.

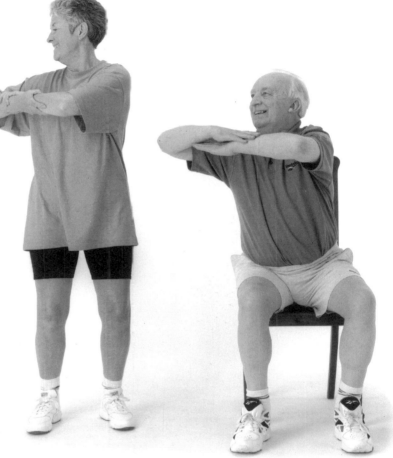

TECHNIQUE TIPS

Keep a firm pelvic tilt to 'fix' the hips forward and prevent the back from arching.

✦

Pause in the centre before turning to the other side.

✦

Make the movements as large as possible; feel them loosening the back, opening the chest.

SEATED ALTERNATIVE

✦ Sit tall with good posture, your legs, feet and arms as for standing, your knees directly over your ankles. Keeping both thighs firmly on the seat, turn to one side as for the standing version above. Return to start position and repeat to other side.

REPEAT 4 TIMES.

N.B. DAILY DOZEN no 5

Warm-up

Low clap swing warmer

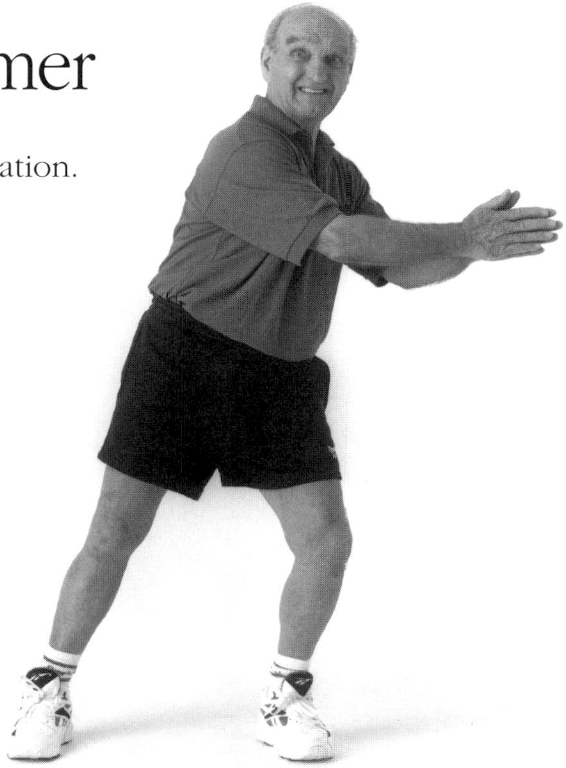

PURPOSE

To warm the muscles and promote circulation.

PREPARATION

✦ Stand tall with good posture, your feet shoulder width apart and toes pointing slightly outwards, knees soft (not locked), abdominals tight to support your back, hands on your hips.

ACTION

✦ Keeping hips facing forward, bend your right knee and transfer your weight to your right side, leaving the left leg straight. Keeping both knees soft, transfer the weight to your left side. Keep the bent knee over the toes and the chest lifted. Go from side to side; build to a comfortable rhythm.

✦ Then, as you bend the right knee sideways, swing both arms across the body to the right side and clap at waist height in front of the body.

✦ Repeat to the left side.

✦ Build to a comfortable rhythm.

CONTINUE FOR 30 SECONDS.

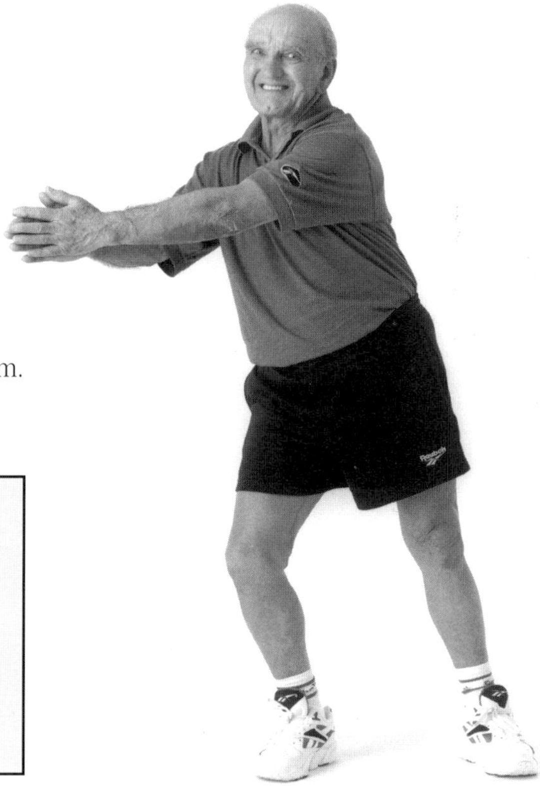

TECHNIQUE TIPS

Enjoy the swinging action but move your arms with control.

✦

Find a rhythm that suits your body and keep your breathing easy and regular.

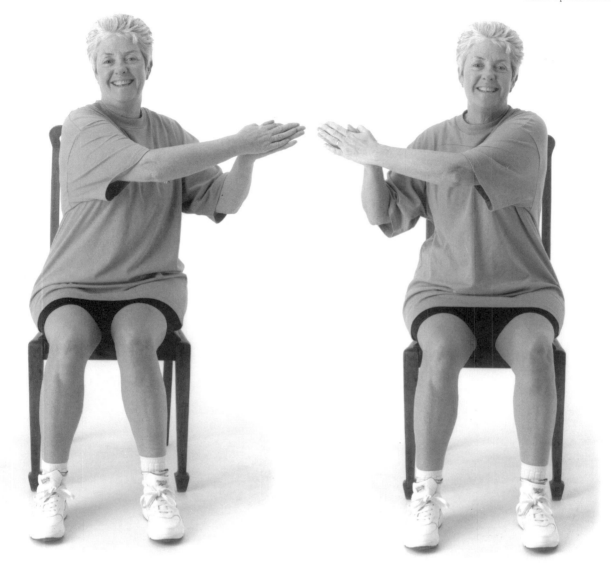

SEATED ALTERNATIVE
- ✦ Sit tall with good posture, legs shoulder width apart and your knees over your ankles. Keeping both thighs firmly on the seat, perform the clapping action at waist level, leaning the body sideways into the movement.

Pelvic rock and roll

PURPOSE

These exercises loosen the lower back, release tension and can ease back pain.

Pelvic rock

PREPARATION

Stand or sit tall with good posture, legs, feet and knees hip width apart. Place both palms on your hips.

ACTION

✦ Do an exaggerated pelvic tilt (see page 55) curving your bottom even further under and pulling your hip bones up towards your nose.

✦ Gradually uncurl the spine until you are back to the starting position. Build this into a gentle rocking motion. Use the hands at first, to emphasise the movement and when you have mastered it, place them on your thighs. Avoid arching your back. Keep the chest lifted and back and neck lengthened.

REPEAT 4 TIMES.

Alternate with pelvic roll (opposite).

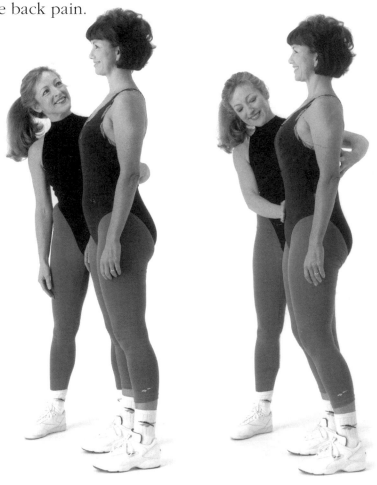

TECHNIQUE TIPS

Feel the movement in your hips and spine.

✦

Move with control and care, keeping your breathing even.

✦

Sitting tall can be tiring for the back. Use this exercise throughout your FITNESS FOR LIFE programme to release tension in the back when it tires.

✦

For the seated alternative support your back by holding the chair seat from time to time.

SEATED ALTERNATIVE

✦ Sit tall. Placing your hands on your thighs, follow the instructions as for the standing version opposite. As you roll down your hands remain in place.

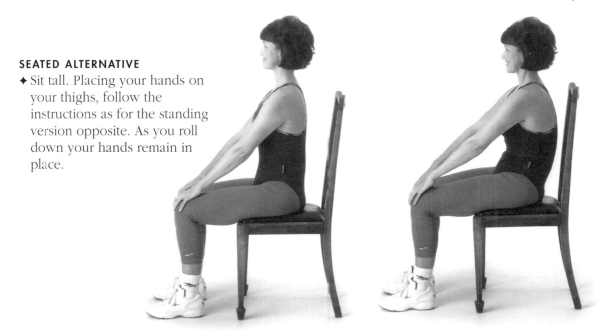

Pelvic rolls

PREPARATION

✦ Stand or sit tall with good posture, your legs and arms as for the pelvic rocks, both feet flat on the floor. Do a pelvic tilt and tighten your tummy muscles. Keeping the spine long and chest lifted, take both hips to the right side, lifting the left hip up towards your right ribs so that you shorten the waist on the right side. Avoid dropping the ribs as you lift hips. Take the hips back to the centre. Repeat to the left side.

✦ Once you have mastered this, place the arms down by your sides and build to a smooth, continuous rolling action from side to side.

REPEAT 8 TIMES.

Alternate with the Pelvic Rock.

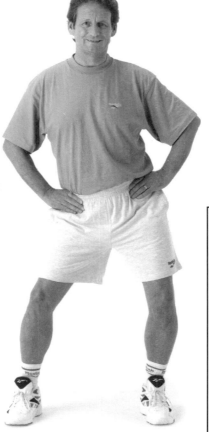

TECHNIQUE TIPS

Keep the knees bent over the ankles, the weight centred between the legs and feet on the floor throughout.

✦

Keep the shoulders over the hips.

✦

Feel the movement in the hips and lower spine.

✦

Keep the breathing easy and the movement controlled.

Ankle activators

PURPOSE

To mobilise the ankles, prevent or reduce stiffness, and improve stability and balance.

PREPARATION

+ Stand tall with good posture, near a wall or the back of a chair for support, your legs and feet about 3 inches apart.

ACTION

+ Bend your knees and centre the weight evenly between your legs. Then transfer the weight to one leg, bending that knee slightly to support your weight. Place the heel of your other foot on the floor, then lift it and place the toes on the floor, in a heel-to-toe action.

+ Repeat 3 to 4 times. Then stand tall and walk on the spot briefly to release any tension.

+ Repeat on the other side.

REPEAT 4 TIMES.

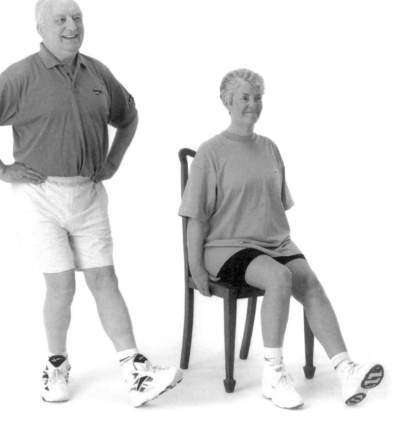

TECHNIQUE TIPS

Keep both knees bent and lift up out of the supporting hip as you do the action.

+

Avoid banging the heel down.

+

Concentrate on increasing the size of the movement at the ankle joint. Try to place the toe on the exact spot where the heel was.

SEATED ALTERNATIVE

If any discomfort is felt in the supporting hip, try this seated alternative. Sit tall with good posture, your ribs lifted and back long, your legs and feet hip width apart and your knees over your ankles. Support your back by holding the chair seat with both hands. Keeping one foot on the floor, put first the heel and then the toes of the other foot on the floor. Try to increase the range of movement by aiming to put the toes directly under the knee.

+ Use the pelvic rock and roll to release any tension (see page 78).

N.B. DAILY DOZEN no 6

Arm circles

PURPOSE

To mobilise the shoulder joints and improve posture.

PREPARATION

✦ Stand or sit tall with good posture, feet hip width apart, knees over your ankles and toes pointing forward.

ACTION

✦ Do a pelvic tilt and tighten the abdominals firmly. Keeping both your hips and shoulders facing front, take one arm forwards to shoulder level, pause, take it upwards until it is close to your ear, pause, and then take it backwards and downwards to the starting position. Avoid arching your back. Now move through each direction in a continuous circle.

✦ Repeat with the other arm.

REPEAT 4 TIMES.

ALTERNATIVE

✦ Stand or sit tall with good posture, bend one arm and place your hand on your shoulder. Circle your elbow in the same pattern as the full arm circles. Repeat for other arm.

✦ When you feel stronger and can move with good control, for variety try both arms together.

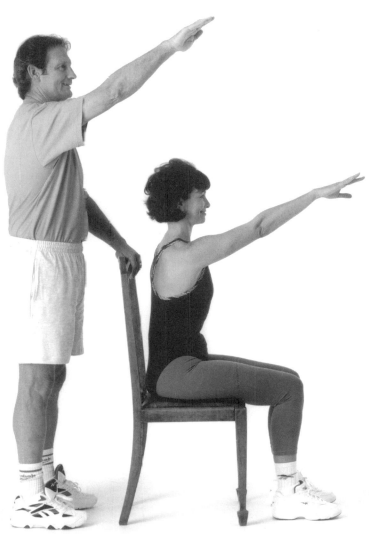

TECHNIQUE TIPS

Take care not to allow your hips or shoulders to turn.

✦

Check your abdominals are tight and avoid arching your back.

✦

Keep the active shoulder pressed down away from your ear.

✦

Keep breathing naturally throughout.

CAUTION

If there is any discomfort in the shoulder at either the forwards or upward position simply make a circle at a height that feels comfortable, or repeat the shoulder circles (page 71).

Knee and hip mobiliser

PURPOSE

This loosens the joints of the hips and knees improves balance and relieves stiffness after long periods of sitting.

PREPARATION

✦ Stand tall with good posture, with or without support, legs hip width apart, knees soft and feet pointing forwards. Centre the weight between your legs. Keep a firm pelvic tilt and tighten the abdominals.

ACTION

✦ Keeping the toes in contact with the floor, lift the heel and ball of one foot off the floor as you bend the knee and lift it upwards. Return heel to the floor. Then alternate legs and gradually build up the size and rhythm of the movement, until the whole foot is coming off the floor, and the knee is lifting as high as is comfortable.

REPEAT 8 TIMES.

SEATED ALTERNATIVE

✦ Sit tall with good posture, your knees bent, hip width apart over your ankles. Hold your chair seat with both hands, and do a firm pelvic tilt and tighten the tummy muscles to support your back.

✦ Perform as for standing version (above) – building gradually to the knee lift. Observe all technique points as before, taking particular care to keep your back long and supported.

TECHNIQUE TIPS

Make sure your chest is lifted and you are standing tall throughout.

✦

Always bring the knee towards the chest and not the chest towards the knee.

✦

If you perform without the support, move your arms in opposition to assist with balance. If you have any balance or joint problems keep the toes of the lifting leg on the floor and use the support until you are stronger.

Neck mobilisers

PURPOSE

To maintain the small but vital movements at the top of the spine
and release neck tension.

PREPARATION

✦ Stand or sit tall with
good posture, look
straight ahead and
lengthen the back of
your neck upwards by
taking the crown of your
head towards the ceiling.
Ease your shoulders
down.

ACTION

✦ Turn your head and look
over your shoulder,
keeping your jaw parallel
with the floor. Hold for a
second and return to the
starting position.
Lengthen your neck and
repeat to the other side.

REPEAT 4 TIMES.

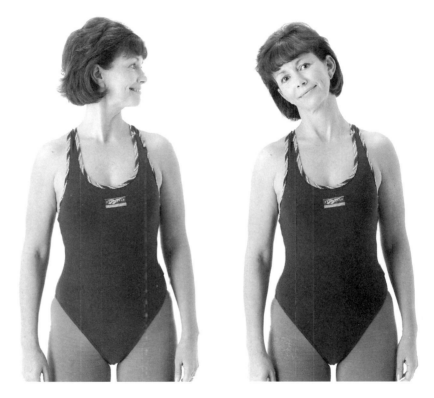

TECHNIQUE TIPS

Do this exercise towards the end of the warm up,
when muscles are more pliable and shoulders less
tense.

✦

Breathe evenly throughout.

✦

Perform all neck moves carefully. Avoid any neck
moves that involve dropping the head backwards.

ALTERNATIVE

✦ Lengthen your neck as before (see picture on
right), and tilt your head and ear towards your
right shoulder. Hold for a second and lift your
head back to the centre. Lengthen and repeat
to the other side.

WARM UP STRETCHES

Inner thigh stretch

PURPOSE

To stretch the inner thigh muscles (adductors) and to improve your performance and reduce injury in every day actions such as walking, climbing on to buses.

PREPARATION

✦ Stand tall, with or without support, with good posture, chest lifted, your legs shoulder width apart, feet pointing slightly outwards, hands on hips.

ACTION

✦ Bend your right knee and keep your left leg straight, weight distributed as evenly as possible between both legs. Keep both hips facing forwards and both feet flat on the ground. Turn the foot of your left leg forward to prevent your ankle rolling in. Feel a mild stretch along your left inner thigh.

✦ Hold for a count of 8 then come back to the centre. Repeat on the other side.

SEATED ALTERNATIVE

✦ Sit tall with good posture, placing your palms on your thighs. Place the soles of your feet together or on the floor wider than shoulder width apart. Allow your knees to fall outward, and press the thighs open until you feel a mild stretch along the inner thigh. Hold for a count of 8, keeping your back long.

CAUTION

Do not do the seated alternative with the feet together if you have had hip surgery or have severe arthritis in the hip or knee joints.

TECHNIQUE TIPS

If standing keep the bent knee over the toe and keep the straight-leg knee soft and facing forwards.

✦

If you cannot feel the stretch, begin again from a wider start position. If the stretch is too strong, narrow the start position.

Calf stretch

PURPOSE

To stretch the muscles of the upper calf (gastrocnemius) and to help lengthen your stride.

PREPARATION

✦ Stand tall with good posture, feet hip width apart.

ACTION

✦ Keeping the width, step one leg backwards and check that the heel and toe of both feet are facing forward; your front knee is bent over your toes.

✦ Ease your weight forward and upward until you feel a mild stretch in the middle of the back of your lower leg.

✦ Keep your back long throughout.

✦ Hold the stretch for a count of 8. Step the back leg in and repeat on the other side.

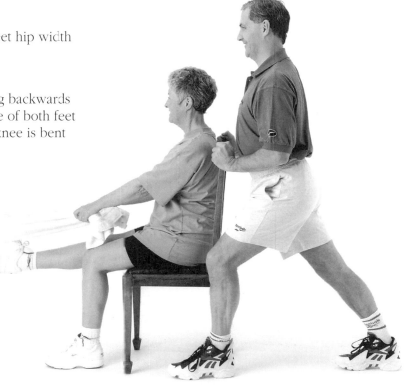

SEATED ALTERNATIVE

✦ Sit tall with good posture, one knee bent and directly above the ankle, the other leg straight out in front with heel resting on floor. Loop a towel round the toes and ball of the foot and hold it firmly in both hands. Lengthen your back and lift your straight leg a little way off the ground. Flex the ankle of your straight leg, bringing the toe towards the shin; pull gently with the towel as you push your heel away until you feel a stretch in the middle of the calf. Hold and repeat as before.

TECHNIQUE TIPS

If balancing is difficult, check that your legs are hip width apart or use a support for effective stretching.

✦

If you cannot feel the stretch, take the back leg a little further back.

✦

Ease gradually into and out of the stretch. Keep your breathing regular to assist stretching.

Lower calf stretch

PURPOSE

To stretch the muscles of the lower calf (soleus) and to put a spring in your step!

PREPARATION

Start as for the calf stretch (see page 83), your feet hip width apart and your front leg bent, your back leg straight and your weight over the front knee.

ACTION

✦ Transfer your weight backwards until it is in the middle of both legs, slightly straightening your front knee and bending the back knee as much as you comfortably can.

✦ Keep the weight in the front of the back foot. Ease downwards into the position until you feel a stretch in the lower calf. If you can't get this stretch at first, keep practising – it's subtle.

✦ Hold the stretch for a count of 8. Repeat for the other calf.

TECHNIQUE TIPS

Take care not to arch the back, and think tall even though the knees are bent.

✦

Keep the back knee over the foot and the heel on the floor.

✦

If balancing is difficult, use a support.

SEATED ALTERNATIVE 1

✦ Sit tall with good posture, one knee bent and directly over the ankle, the other knee taken back under the chair as far as possible with the ball of the foot on the floor and heel raised. Press this heel towards the floor until you feel a stretch in the base of the calf. Hold and repeat as before.

SEATED ALTERNATIVE 2

✦ As seated alternative in the calf stretch (see page 83) but this time slightly bending the leg being stretched with the towel.

Top of thigh stretch

PURPOSE

To stretch the muscles that bend
the hip (hip flexors) to increase
range of hip movement and
reduce stiffness.

PREPARATION

✦ Start as for the calf stretch, standing
tall with good posture, your legs hip
width apart and feet facing forward,
your front knee bent, your back leg
straight and your weight over front
knee.

ACTION

✦ Bend your back knee slightly and
do an exaggerated pelvic tilt to
bring your hips up towards your
nose.

✦ Lift up out of your hips,
lengthening your upper body
backwards and upwards; then
re-tilt the pelvis. You will
feel a mild stretch in the
front of the hip of your
back leg.

✦ Hold for a count of 8.
Rest actively by doing
the Pelvic Roll (page
76) from the Warm
Up.

✦ Repeat on the
opposite side.

A seated alternative
s on page 87.

TECHNIQUE TIPS

Keep both hips facing front.
✦
Keep abdominals tight for an
effective stretch.
✦
Use a support for stability.
✦
Ease gradually into and out of
the stretch, breathing naturally
and regularly.

Front of thigh stretch

PURPOSE

To stretch the muscles at the front of the thigh (quadriceps), improve hip movement and counteract the shortening effects of sitting.

PREPARATION

✦ Stand tall with good posture, facing the support of a wall or chair, your legs together and feet facing forward, your hands resting on the support.

ACTION

✦ Bend both knees slightly and transfer your weight on to the left leg as you bring your right knee up towards your chest.

✦ Keeping the abdominals tight and back long,

take hold of the back (or front) of your right ankle (or sock) and take this bent leg back until the thigh and knee are behind the hip. Take care not to arch your back. You will feel a strong stretch down the front of your right thigh. Re-tilt the pelvis if you need to increase the stretch.

✦ Hold for a count of 8. Release the leg to the floor with extra control. Circle the hips to relieve any tension.

✦ **REPEAT FOR THE OTHER LEG.**

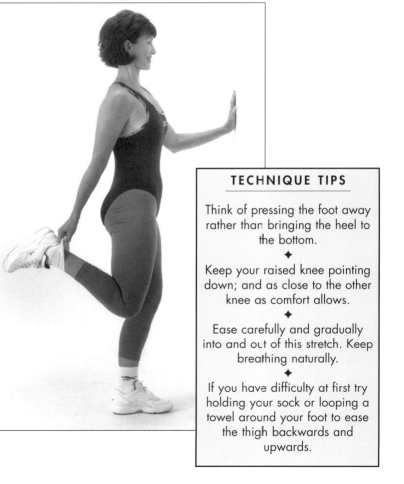

TECHNIQUE TIPS

Think of pressing the foot away rather than bringing the heel to the bottom.

✦

Keep your raised knee pointing down; and as close to the other knee as comfort allows.

✦

Ease carefully and gradually into and out of this stretch. Keep breathing naturally.

✦

If you have difficulty at first try holding your sock or looping a towel around your foot to ease the thigh backwards and upwards.

SEATED ALTERNATIVE

✦ Sit tall with good posture, sideways on the chair, both feet flat on the floor. Support yourself with one arm on the back of the chair. Keeping both hips facing forward, move your right leg carefully backwards along the front of the chair until your thigh and knee are behind the hip. Re-tilt your pelvis and feel the stretch as before. Hold for a count of 8.

CAUTION

✦ In the standing version, if you experience any discomfort in the bent knee, in the standing version, try holding the leg a little more to the side. If discomfort persists, come out of the stretch, miss this exercise and repeat the front of hip stretch.

✦ If you experience cramp in the back of the thigh as you take the leg back, try the seated or towel alternative or leave this exercise until your circulation and general muscle tone have improved.

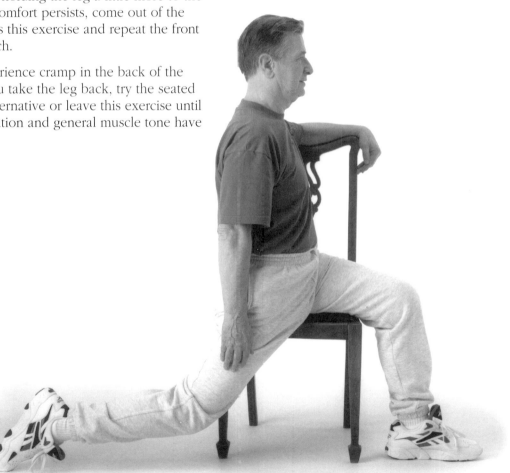

Warm-up

Upward side stretch

PURPOSE

To stretch the muscles at the side of the trunk (latissimus dorsi), improve your posture and keep your body tall.

PREPARATION

Stand with your feet shoulder width apart, knees slightly bent and the toes pointing forward. Place one hand on your hip to support the back and lift the other arm up to the ceiling.

ACTION

✦ Do a pelvic tilt, tighten the abdominals and really extend your arm and trunk upwards, then very slightly sideways over the crown of your head. Take care not to arch the back. Keep the extended arm in line with the ear so you are not leaning forwards or backwards. Feel a stretch down the left side of the body and ribs.

✦ Hold for a count of 8 and then repeat the stretch again. Release, rest and repeat on the other side.

SEATED ALTERNATIVE 1

✦ Sit tall with good posture, your legs shoulder width apart and knees over your ankles. Place one hand on the chair seat or your hip for support and reach up with the other arm as for the standing stretch.

ALTERNATIVE 2

✦ If you have difficulty with arm movements above the shoulder, either bend your arm and placing your hand on your shoulder lead the stretch with your elbow instead or keep both arms at your sides and perform the trunk move as above.

TECHNIQUE TIPS

Keep both shoulders down, knees bent and weight even between both feet.

✦

Stretch upwards not sideways.

✦

Ease gradually into and out of the stretch. Keep breathing evenly and naturally.

N.B. DAILY DOZEN no 8

Chest stretch

PURPOSE

To stretch the muscles across the front of the chest (pectorals), improve your lung capacity and tone your upper back. This also gives you an immediate release of energy.

PREPARATION

✦ Stand or sit tall with good posture, your legs hip width apart and toes pointing forwards. Palms resting lightly on your bottom.

ACTION

✦ Tightening your abdominals to prevent your lower back from arching, draw the elbows and shoulder blades together at the back until you feel a stretch across the front of your chest, the tops of your shoulders and arms.

✦ Hold the stretch for a count of 8. Release the arms, circle the shoulders and repeat the stretch.

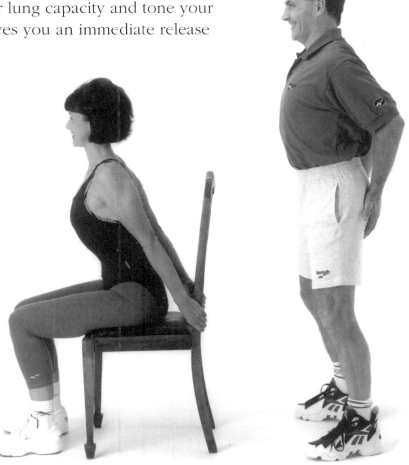

TECHNIQUE TIPS

Keep the back of your neck long, jaw parallel with the floor, your chest lifted and tummy pulled in.

✦

Ease gradually into and out of the stretch. Breathe evenly throughout.

SEATED ALTERNATIVE

✦ Sit tall with good posture. Take your arms backwards and hold on to the back of the chair with both hands. Lean forwards and upwards, letting your arms lengthen and straighten against the weight of your body until you feel the stretch across your chest. Hold and repeat as before.

N.B. DAILY DOZEN no 9

Back-of-thigh stretch

PURPOSE

To stretch the muscles at the back of the thigh (hamstrings) and maintain a good range of movement at the hip.

PREPARATION

Sit tall with good posture, near the edge of your chair, legs hip width apart and knees bent over the ankles.

ACTION

✦ Straighten one leg out in front of you, resting your heel on the floor. Place both hands just above the bent knee to support your back and body weight. Lift the chest and lengthen the whole upper body upwards and forwards until you feel a stretch in the back of the straight thigh.

✦ Hold for a count of 8; release and repeat on the other side.

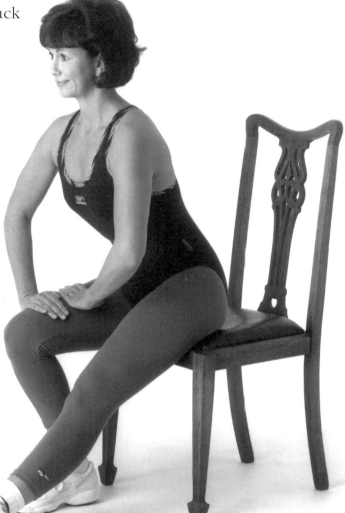

TECHNIQUE TIPS

If you can't feel the stretch, try tilting your bottom upwards a little but avoid arching your back.

✦

If you feel the stretch in the calf, take your toe nearer to the floor.

✦

Ease gradually into and out of the stretch. Keep breathing even.

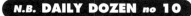

N.B. **DAILY DOZEN** *no* **10**

Back-of-arm stretch

PURPOSE

To stretch the muscles at the back of the arm (triceps) and increase the range of movement in the shoulder joints.

PREPARATION

+ Sit or stand tall with good posture, your feet and legs hip width apart and knees bent.

ACTION

+ Lift your right arm up to the ceiling and bend the elbow bringing your fingers as far down your back as possible. Take left arm across your chest and support the raised right arm with your left hand. Ease right arm up and back until you feel a stretch along the underside of the arm.

+ Hold for a count of 8. Release, circle the shoulder. Repeat on the other arm.

ALTERNATIVES

+ Stand or sit tall with good posture. Holding a towel in your right arm lift it to the ceiling and bend the elbow so that the towel hangs down your back. Taking your left arm around your back and, holding as far up the opposite end of the towel as possible, gently draw your right arm down, until you feel the stretch.

+ If you have difficulty with arm movements above the shoulder, try taking the right arm as far across the chest as possible so that it is lying across the bend of the left arm. Bend the left arm up and gently ease the right arm into the chest until you feel a stretch in the top of the right arm.

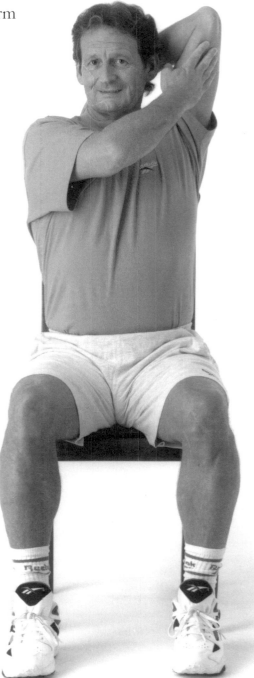

Stamina Conditioning Plan

STAMINA CONDITIONING WORKOUT: 10 TO 20 MINUTES

The purpose of all aerobic exercises is to condition the heart, lungs and muscles, and to increase circulation, stamina and energy. The Fitness For Life exercises are lively and fun to perform. They use travelling, swinging, rhythmical moves that will make you breathe more heavily and your heart beat more strongly and quickly. You will find yourself getting really warm and probably perspiring a little. Always try the talk test. If you are finding the exercises too hard and becoming so breathless that you can't talk, make the movements smaller and stop using the arms. You will soon feel more comfortable and ready to go again. NEVER stop suddenly in the stamina section; always wind down gradually. If you can talk too easily, work a little harder – making the moves bigger and deeper.

The stamina workout begins with the Easy Walks 1 and 2 from the Warm Up (page 69), and progresses to the more vigorous pace of Bodywalks 1, 2 and 3 here. Remember that once you've started this aerobic section, there is no stopping! It is important to vary the pace to suit you, but the legs should move continuously, for safe and effective training. If you do these exercises regularly you will find your heart and lungs get fit very quickly and breathlessness will be a thing of the past. The stamina workout climbs gradually with body-warming moves that **build up** in aerobic pace and size to a level that is comfortably hard – the **maintenance** stage. This is sustained for a target time before the **aerobic cool down** begins and progresses slowly down to where the stamina section started. Make sure you follow this safety route, alternating bursts of energy with a 'moderately does it' approach on the way. And if you're feeling less than energetic and this doesn't change after the build up stamina section then an 'easy does it' approach is the best for that day.

Once you are familiar with these moves, start to put more effort into them. Travel, use the space and really enjoy yourself.

STAMINA (AEROBIC EXERCISES)

Bodywalk 1

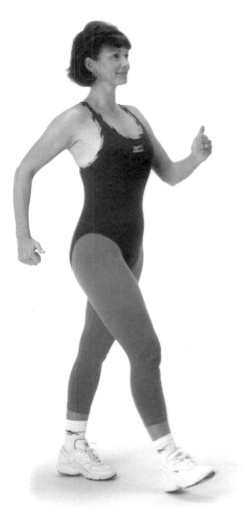

PREPARATION

✦ Stand with good posture, your legs and feet about 3 inches apart and your toes facing forward as for Easy Walk 1 and 2 (see page 69).

ACTION

✦ Begin by doing 30 seconds of on-the-spot Easy Walk 1 bringing in any low, swinging arm action, that feels natural, without stopping. Progress to Easy Walk 2 for 30 seconds travelling at a moderate strolling pace.

✦ Consciously step up the pace to a brisker walk. Transfer your weight on each step with a heel-through-to-toe rolling action. Lengthen your stride a little and walk tall. The arms bend at the elbow, close to the body, the forearms and palms face inwards, thumbs on top; they swing backwards and forwards at waist level.

✦ Continue for 30 seconds more. Repeat from the top with bigger moves and more energy.

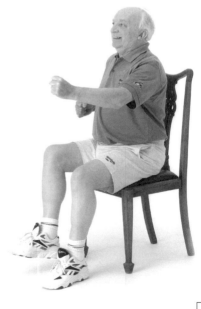

SEATED ALTERNATIVE

PREPARATION

✦ Sit tall with good posture, your legs and feet hip width apart and your knees over your ankles. Begin by doing 30 seconds of EASYWALK 1 (page 69) with large marching arm actions, your elbows bent, palms in and swinging loosely. Progress to EASYWALK 2 (page 69) for 30 seconds.

ACTION

✦ Sit tall with good posture, tighten the abdominals secure your back, and lift your bent legs alternately in a relaxed marching action. Swing your arms strongly through at waist level.

✦ Continue for 30 seconds or until your legs begin to tire. Take each leg out in front alternately in a loose toe tapping action, to release tension in the legs.

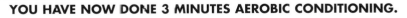

YOU HAVE NOW DONE 3 MINUTES AEROBIC CONDITIONING.

Stamina Conditioning Plan

Bodywalk 2

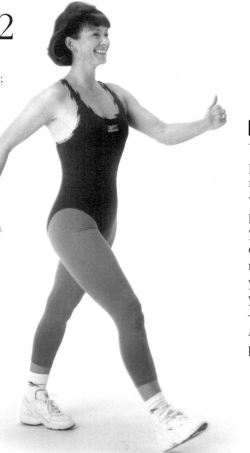

ACTION

✦ Lengthen your stride again; push through the balls of your feet more and quicken the pace to a really brisk walk. Take your elbows further back and swing them further so the arms make more of a 'driving through' action.

✦ Build to a rhythm and a speed that feels natural for your body.

✦ Continue for 30 seconds. Repeat from the beginning (Easy Walk 1 and 2, Bodywalk 1 and 2) with even more energy now you have got into your stride.

CAUTION

You will get warmer and perspire; your heart will beat more quickly, your breathing will be heavier and you will be puffing harder than usual; but you should feel comfortable enough to count out loud and move with energy. If you find you are gasping for breath, or your legs or arms feel like lead – you are working far too hard. Adjust your effort by easing the pace.

SEATED ALTERNATIVE

Sit tall and increase the pace of the march and the height of your knee lift. Your arms increase in pace taking your elbow back further and driving through further each time.

✦ Continue for 30 seconds or until your legs begin to tire.

✦ Alternate the march with the toe tapping action to the front, until you have completed another 3 minutes

---

YOU HAVE NOW DONE 6 MINUTES OF AEROBIC EXERCISE.
✦ To continue the AEROBIC CONDITIONING, PROGRESS TO BODYWALK 3.
✦ If you are doing THE MINI WORKOUT or THE MUSCLE CONDITIONING WORKOUT continue with the AEROBIC COOL DOWN (see page 101).
✦ To progress UP in aerobic pace go to BODYWALK 3. To proceed to something a little more easy, return to BODYWALK 1. To maintain the pace, stay with BODYWALK 2.

Bodywalk 3

ACTION

◆ Increase the pace again and very slightly shorten your stride. The arms take on more of a pumping action as you maintain the backward move of the elbow but shorten the drive through, so increasing the speed and number of arm swings to complement the shorter strides. Check your posture frequently. A pelvic tilt, long back and tight abdominals are essential to stabilise your back and prevent your hips rolling.

◆ Do this for 1 minute, then alternate it with BODYWALK 2 (or one of the other stamina exercises that follow) for a further 3 minutes.

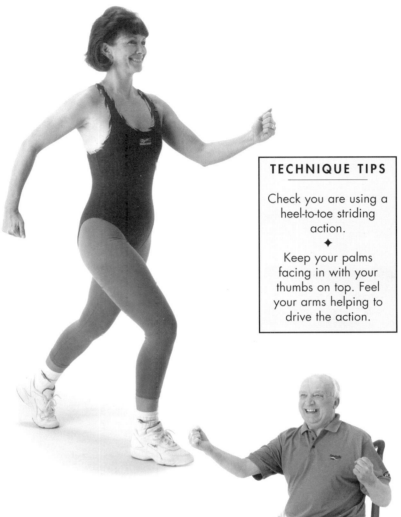

TECHNIQUE TIPS

Check you are using a heel-to-toe striding action.

◆

Keep your palms facing in with your thumbs on top. Feel your arms helping to drive the action.

SEATED ALTERNATIVE

ACTION

◆ Sit tall and perform a really slow, controlled march. As you lift each knee up, lift both your arms out in front, or up to the ceiling, bring them down to the hips and lift them again on the next knee lift.

◆ Continue for 30 seconds or until your legs or arms begin to tire. Alternate with toe taps as before.

YOU HAVE DONE 8 MINUTES OF AEROBIC EXERCISE
If you have had enough for today, proceed to the AEROBIC COOL DOWN (see page 101).
If you wish to continue to the MAINTENANCE AEROBIC CONDITIONING stage, turn to the next page.

MAINTENANCE AEROBIC CONDITIONING
High clap swing warmer

PREPARATION
+ As for slow clap swing warmer (see page 74)

ACTION
+ Begin with your legs and feet shoulder width apart, clapping from side to side, as for LOW CLAP SWING WARMER, until you get back into the rhythm.

+ Then make the moves bigger, deepening the knee bends and clapping high right, high left, low left and low right, until you are clapping a big square in the air in front of your body.

+ Continue for 30 seconds, then BODY WALK 1, 2 or 3 for 30 seconds (see pages 93–95).

TECHNIQUE TIPS

Keep the back long, stabilising it with a pelvic tilt and tight abdominals when using your arms.

✦

Keep all arm moves controlled and in front of the body to avoid twisting.

✦

Work within your limitations: 'comfortably challenged' but no more. If you find you are gasping for breath, exhausted, overheated or uncomfortable in any way, keep the legs moving but stop using your arms and make the moves smaller until you recover.

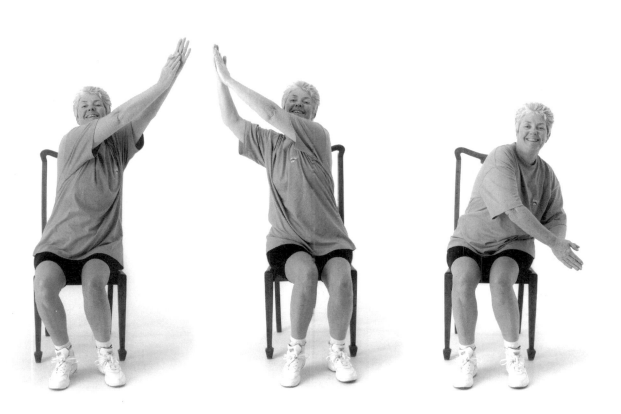

SEATED ALTERNATIVE 1

✦ Sit tall with good posture, your legs shoulder width apart or wider for stability, knees over the ankles, feet pointing slightly outwards and flat on the floor. Complete exercise as opposite.

SEATED ALTERNATIVE 2

✦ Proceed to an easier pace with the original LOW CLAP SWING WARMER (see page 74) if you feel this is a better option.

TO PROGRESS

✦ Progress the standing version by rising up on the toes on the high moves or even rising up onto the toes of the outside foot and taking the other leg off the floor in a small balance if you feel confident and controlled.

Canoeing step tap

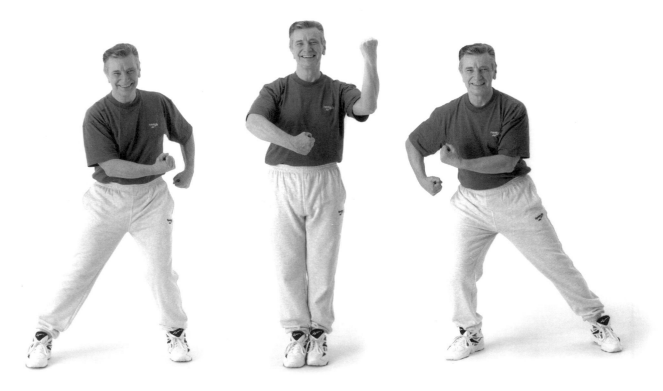

PREPARATION

◆ Stand tall with good posture, your feet and legs together, feet facing forward and knees slightly bent, your hands on your hips.

ACTION

◆ Step right foot sideways to take the weight as you bring the left foot next to the instep of the right foot and tap it on the floor. Immediately repeat to the left side. Both knees stay over the toes, slightly bent throughout. Repeat to the left side. Repeat the moves, building them into a rhythm and enlarging the actions by standing tall as the feet come together and deepening the knee bends on the taps.

◆ The rhythmical arm actions are just like paddling a canoe. Hold the imaginary paddle upright in front of your chest. As you take the step to the right, paddle to the right (left hand

> ### TECHNIQUE TIPS
>
> Keep the chest lifted and stand tall on the knee bends.
>
> ◆
>
> Feel 'comfortably challenged' and no more. If you find you are gasping for breath, exhausted, overheated or uncomfortable in any way – adjust your effort.

on top and right underneath). Step the left foot in and bring the paddle upright (right hand on top), left underneath. Repeat to the left. Build to a rhythm that suits you. If you don't enjoy the canoeing action – anything goes! As long as you keep moving.

◆ Continue for 30 seconds then BODY WALK 1, 2 or 3 (pages 93–95) for 30 seconds.

SEATED ALTERNATIVE 1

◆ Sit tall with good posture, your legs and feet close together, knees over your ankles, heels lifted up, and your weight resting on the balls of the feet. Complete as for standing.

◆ Continue for 30 seconds or until arms or legs tire. Tap the toes alternately on the floor, holding the chair to support your back and release tension in the limbs. Then repeat canoe swings.

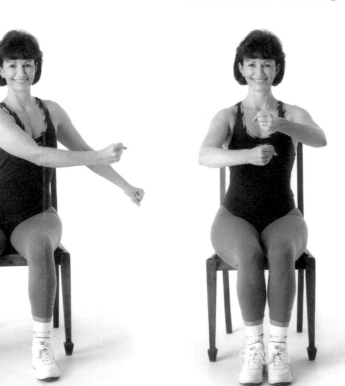

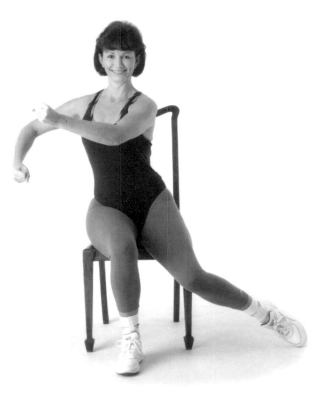

STANDING ALTERNATIVES

◆ To progress the standing version, push right up on the balls of the feet, bend a little deeper, or even take the side step into a small spring. Always bend the knees before and after any jump, no matter how small; and land toe-ball-heel for safety.

◆ **For variety**, you can travel this step forwards and backwards.

◆ To move to an easier pace, perform with your hands on your hips and decrease the size of steps.

N.B. DAILY DOZEN no 9

Ski lifts

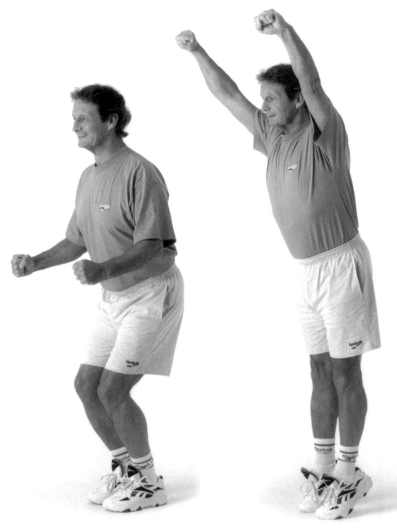

PREPARATION

◆ Stand with good posture, your feet together, knees bent, arms slightly back from the shoulders, elbows bent and palms facing in as if holding ski poles. Lean your weight slightly more forward than usual into the front of your foot.

ACTION

◆ Increase the knee bend and, leading with the arms, extend the legs and lift up onto the balls of your feet as if about to jump into the air. Hold the balance for a moment before lowering your arms, bending your knees and repeating the move.

◆ Take 3 walking steps forward and bring the legs together and repeat the 2 ski lifts.

◆ Continue for 30 seconds then BODY WALK 1, 2 or 3 for 30 seconds. Repeat SKI LIFTS and BODY WALK again.

TECHNIQUE TIPS

Take care not to drop the chest when bending the knees, and keep the heels on the floor.

◆

Keep the weight forward and upward, even on the bending moves.

◆

Keep the weight on the big toe when rising on the toes.

◆

Always have bent knees to take off and land. Always land toe, ball, heel.

◆

Work within your limitations and adjust your effort if necessary.

STANDING ALTERNATIVE

◆ To progress in standing build the ski lift into a small spring or jump from 2 feet to 2 feet. You can also use skipping instead of walking to pep up the pace even further.

YOU HAVE NOW DONE 12 MINUTES OF AEROBIC CONDITIONING

If you have done enough for today, proceed to the AEROBIC COOL DOWN (see page opposite). If you wish to go to the 16 MINUTE AEROBIC STAGE continue with the STAMINA/AEROBIC WORKOUT MOVES AND BODY WALK COMBINATIONS (see pages 93–95) FOR A FURTHER 4 MINUTES.

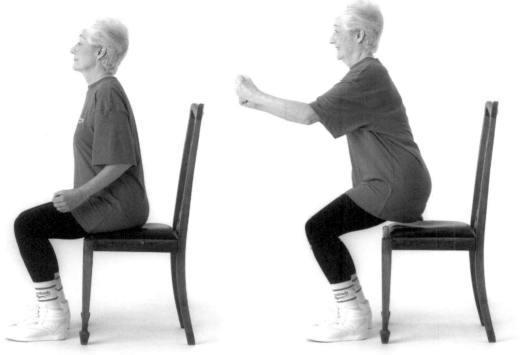

SEATED ALTERNATIVE

✦ Sit tall with good posture. Complete exercise as for standing but marching instead of walking. Really feel your whole body lifting upwards on the 'lift'. Keep the chest lifted and extend the arms in front on the 'take off' and behind on the 'landing'. If possible, progress to lifting the thighs just off the chair, tightening the abdominals and pushing on the thighs. Think of pushing upwards rather than forwards, as if preparing to stand.

YOU HAVE DONE 16 MINUTES OF AEROBIC CONDITIONING

Do a final 30 seconds worth of your favourite move. Then begin your AEROBIC COOL DOWN.

AEROBIC COOL DOWN

1) Your favourite move with low arms for 30 seconds. Then BODY WALK 2 for 30 seconds.

OR

2) Your favourite move with no arms for 30 seconds. Then BODY WALK 2 with low arms for 30 seconds.

OR

3) BODY WALK 1 with no arms for 30 seconds. EASY WALK 2 for 30 seconds.

OR

4) EASY WALK 1 for 30 seconds and continue until you and your body feel completely back to normal, breathing easily and regularly.

MOVING ON

If you are finishing here for today, remember to stretch the calves (pages 83–84), the front, back and inside of the thighs (page 82) to get the full benefits. If you are continuing with the Muscle Conditioning Plan, stretch the calves only, before beginning the muscle fitness exercises.

Muscle Conditioning Plan

MUSCLE FITNESS CONDITIONING (ENDURANCE, STRENGTHENING AND FLEXIBILITY STRETCHING EXERCISES): 20 MINUTES +

Muscular strength and local muscle endurance exercises

These exercises target specific muscle groups, to build strength, power and endurance. They transform posture, straighten rounded shoulders, tighten tummy muscles and firm the arm, legs, hips and pelvic floor muscles. Most importantly, they strengthen bones. Technique is important to ensure safety and results. Take your time getting into position and then work the muscles to the point of overload, but **not** beyond it. When you begin to feel the muscles tire or ache, do one more repetition, then mobilise and rest before beginning again.

If you find it difficult to continue, do not do that exercise again that day. A Body Warming exercise (see pages 69 and 74) and rest will help the muscle to recover quickly. As you improve, add more repetitions or resistance.

Take time to study the technique tips. Always breathe easily in these exercises, as holding your breath can build tension and reduce benefits. And remember it is better to exercise **all the muscles once** rather than concentrate on a few muscles. Then, if you have to miss a day, it doesn't matter so much.

Flexibility stretches

Stretching exercises are essential to gain flexibility for all round fitness and assist your body in returning to its steady state (**cool down**) after the workout sections. The flexibility stretches are more relaxed and, as the muscles are very warm, deeper, **longer** stretches are possible and will develop that all important suppleness. Certain muscles lend themselves to this **developmental** stretching and the best results are seen when this is done daily and repeated three times. The shorter stretches in this section (**maintenance stretching**) return the other muscles to their natural length. Effective stretching is a skill, and comfort is the key. Stretching is very individual, so try out the various alternative positions offered to find which suits you best. If you take time to stretch all the muscles correctly and **comfortably**, feeling the stretch in the bulky part of the muscle, you will feel and look lithe and will protect older, more vulnerable muscles from injury and shortening.

A unique feature of the Fitness for Life Plan is that there are stretches throughout the muscle conditioning section to provide active rests in between the strength exercises. This not only helps you to use each position to the full, but more importantly helps to avoid the tension that may be felt in the older body when the stretches are done all together. The words 'Flexibility Plus' at the top of the page signal the beginning of this mix of stretching and strength and endurance exercises.

STRENGTH AND ENDURANCE EXERCISES

Ankle strengthener

PURPOSE

To condition the muscles in the ankles (flexors and extensors), and strengthen the ankle bones.

PREPARATION

✦ Sit tall with good posture, your thighs together and knees bent, your lower legs and feet several inches apart and slightly forwards. Hold the chair to support your back.

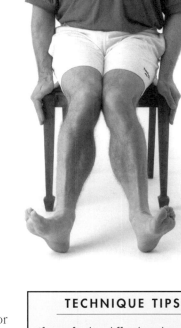

ACTION

✦ Keeping your knees in contact and your heels on the floor, lift both feet inwards and upwards as much as possible. Hold for a second. Then brush both feet outwards along the floor past the start position and lift them up at the end of the move as much as possible. Hold.

✦ Then brush them back along the floor past the start position and lift again.

✦ Repeat as often as you like until the muscles begin to tire. Rest with some Easy Walks (see page 69). As you get fitter, build to a maximum of 12 repetitions in each set.

REPEAT X 1 MORE SET.

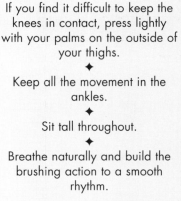

TECHNIQUE TIPS

If you find it difficult to keep the knees in contact, press lightly with your palms on the outside of your thighs.

✦

Keep all the movement in the ankles.

✦

Sit tall throughout.

✦

Breathe naturally and build the brushing action to a smooth rhythm.

Heel raises

PURPOSE

To condition the muscles in the backs of the lower legs (calves – gastrocnemius muscles) and to strengthen the ankle bones.

PREPARATION

✦ Stand tall with good posture, and the support of a wall or chair. Your legs and feet about one inch apart, knees 'soft' and directly over your ankles, elbows slightly bent and just in front of your body, hands resting lightly on the support. Do a firm pelvic tilt and tighten your tummy muscles. Keep ribs lifted and shoulders down. Look straight ahead.

ACTION

✦ Keeping the weight evenly distributed between both feet, lift your heels and body upwards as far as possible by pushing up through the balls of your feet and toes. Hold for a second, then lower your heels so that they just touch down lightly before lifting up again.

✦ Repeat until your legs begin to tire, then do one more and walk on the spot to refresh the muscles. As you get fitter, build up to a maximum of 12 repetitions in each set.

REPEAT X 2 MORE SETS.

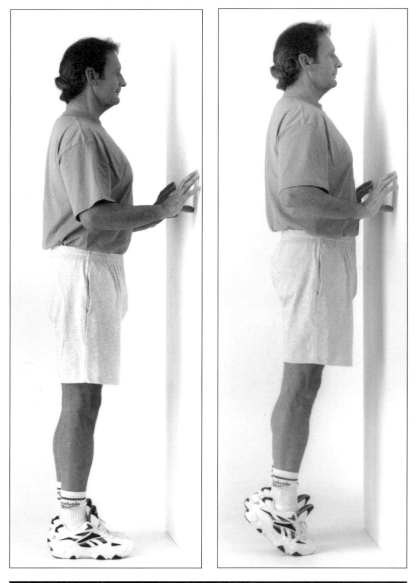

CAUTION

If you have bunions or arthritis in the toe joints, keep your weight where it is most comfortable; if standing, use the support more or choose the seated alternative. Complete just 3 repetitions to start. See how your foot is the next day before continuing.

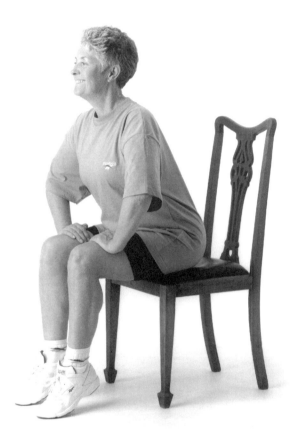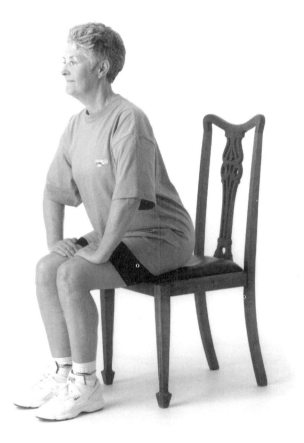

SEATED ALTERNATIVE

✦ Sit tall with good posture, your legs, feet and knees hip width apart. Palms on your thighs, elbows bent.

✦ Perform the exercise as for standing but push down through your thighs and feet to add resistance. Once you have mastered this, lean your body weight slightly forwards and upwards from the hips to add weight.

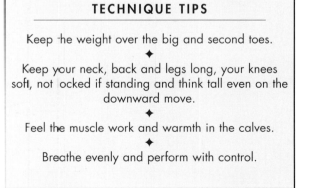

TECHNIQUE TIPS

Keep the weight over the big and second toes.
✦
Keep your neck, back and legs long, your knees soft, not locked if standing and think tall even on the downward move.
✦
Feel the muscle work and warmth in the calves.
✦
Breathe evenly and perform with control.

Stride knee bends

PURPOSE

To condition the muscles at the front and back of the thighs (quadriceps, hamstrings) and buttocks (gluteals). This will strengthen the vulnerable hip bones and improve many daily actions.

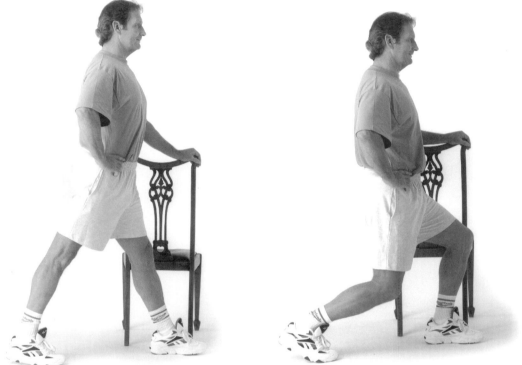

PREPARATION

✦ Stand tall with good posture, side on to a wall or chair for support. Place your legs and feet hip width apart, toes pointing forwards; one arm slightly bent with the palm resting on the support, the other hand on your hip.

ACTION

✦ Keeping your back straight and chest lifted throughout, take one stride length forwards with the leg nearest the support. Your back heel will come off the floor.

✦ Keeping a firm pelvic tilt and tight abdominals, bend both knees and lower your body about 4 inches. Do not bend your knees further. Push

straight up through your feet and thighs, returning to the start. Rest in place for a second.

✦ Repeat until the legs begin to tire. Complete the move and walk on the spot to refresh the muscles. As you get fitter, build up to a maximum of 12 repetitions in each set.

✦ Turn around and repeat on other side.

REPEAT X 2 MORE SETS.

CAUTION

If you have any discomfort in your knees during this exercise do the alternative.

TECHNIQUE TIPS

Keep both knees in line with the toes throughout.

✦

Feel the strength in the thighs as they lift you back to start.

✦

Keep breathing steady and the movement controlled.

ALTERNATIVE

✦ For this 'Sit and Stand' exercise, sit tall with good posture near the front of the chair, your legs and feet hip width apart, heels on the floor and slightly further back than usual, your knees over your toes and palms on your knees. Do a pelvic tilt, tighten your tummy muscles strongly and lean forwards slightly from the hips.

✦ Tighten your thighs as if about to stand. Press down through your thighs and feet as you lift your weight up about an inch. Lower with control back to the start. Keep the head up and spine long throughout. Build this lifting and lowering action up, an inch at a time, until you can stand tall in one swift, controlled move without your hands.

✦ Reverse by lowering slowly one inch at a time until you are one inch from your seat. Lower this last inch with extra control. Feel the muscle work in the thighs and buttocks. Then sit back and enjoy your new strength for a moment before continuing.

REPEAT AS FOR STANDING.

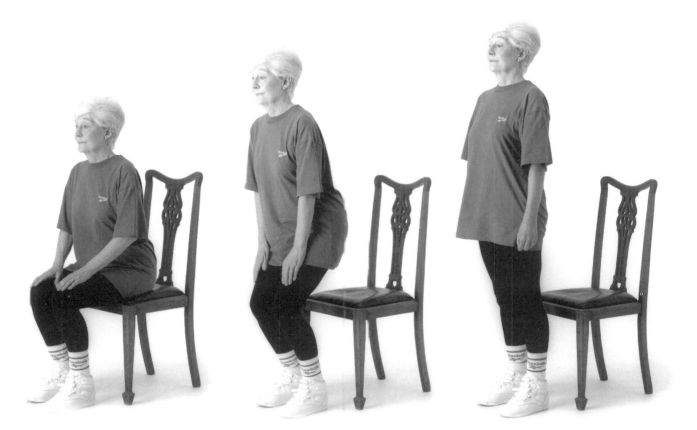

Wall press up

PURPOSE

To condition the muscles at the back of the arm (triceps) and chest (pectorals) and to strengthen the bones of the shoulders and arms.

PREPARATION

♦ Stand tall with good posture, facing a wall. Place your palms on the wall just wider than shoulder width apart and walk your feet backwards several inches. Adjust your feet so they are hip width apart and facing forwards, your arms straight, elbows and knees soft. Increase the pelvic tilt and tighten the abdominals.

ACTION

♦ Bend your elbows, lowering your body towards the wall. Press firmly against the wall to return to the start position. Take care not to let your back sag; keep it long, and your abdominals tight, throughout.

♦ Repeat until the arms begin to tire. Rest by circling the shoulders and wrists. As you get fitter, build to a maximum of 12 repetitions in each set.

REPEAT X 2 MORE SETS.

♦ **For variety:** Once you are stronger, add a 'free fall' movement. As you push back, push away so your hands come off the wall a couple of inches. 'Drop' back onto the wall, using smooth control as before.

♦ You may prefer to use the 'box' position (see page 57).

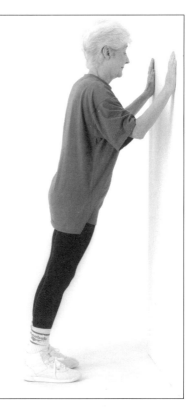
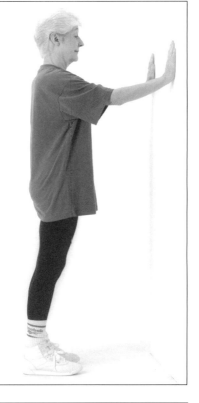

TECHNIQUE TIPS

Take the top of your forehead, not your nose, towards the wall.

♦

Avoid locking the elbows as you return to the start.

♦

Feel the muscle work in the back of the upper arms and across the chest.

♦

Try breathing out as you push away, but find your own breathing rhythm if this doesn't work for you.

CAUTION

If there is any strain in the shoulder joint, or one side seems weaker, make the lowering action smaller and narrow the hands a little.

If there is any discomfort in your wrists during this exercise, because of stiffness, arthritis or other problems, try the backward press (opposite).

Backward press

PURPOSE

To condition the muscles at the back of the arm (triceps) and upper back (trapezius) and strengthen the spine and shoulder bones.

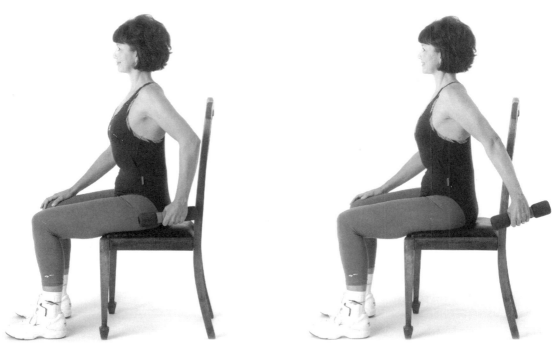

PREPARATION

✦ Sit or stand tall with good posture, with or without weights. Position your legs, knees and feet hip width apart; one arm on your thigh, the other at your side with the weight, if used, held securely in your palm. Take the arm back as far as possible and bend the elbow so that the forearm hangs down at right angles, palm (and weight) facing backwards. Avoid arching the back by keeping the spine and neck long, and the abdominals tight.

ACTION

✦ Straighten your forearm taking your hand (and weight) to the ceiling, taking care not to lock the elbows. Lower to the right angle position.

✦ Repeat until arm (or upper back) tires. Build up to a maximum of 12. Rest. Circle your shoulders to release any tension. Repeat with other arm.

REPEAT X 2 MORE SETS.

TECHNIQUE TIPS

Keep the upper arms close to the body, and the chest lifted away from the waist.

✦

Feel the muscles work at the back of the arms and in the upper back.

✦

Keep breathing natural and regular, and the movement slow and controlled.

ALTERNATIVE

✦ Perform without weights, or progress to a heavier weight as appropriate.

Thigh Strengthener

PURPOSE

To condition the thigh muscles (quadriceps), stabilise the knee joint and strengthen the hip.

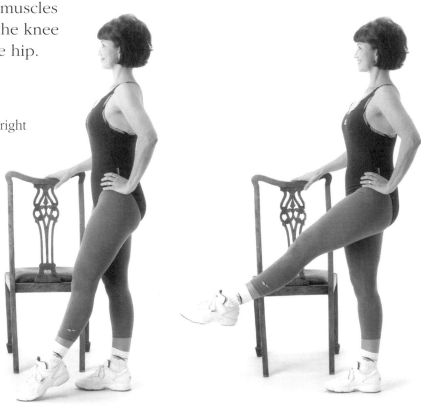

PREPARATION

✦ Stand tall with good posture right side on to a wall or chair for support, knees and toes pointing forward; right elbow slightly bent, palm resting on the support just above waist level, the left hand on the hip. Increase the pelvic tilt and tighten your tummy muscles.

ACTION

✦ Lift up out of both hips and then, resting your toes on the ground, slide the left leg forward.

✦ Tighten the thigh muscles and keep the knee straight as you lengthen and then lift your leg about 3 inches, hold for a second, then return it to the floor. Rest for a second. Check the posture, centre the weight, and repeat until the leg tires, then do one more repetition and circle the hips to release tension. Build to a maximum of 8.

✦ Turn around and repeat with other leg.

REPEAT X 2 MORE SETS.

CAUTION

If this exercise causes discomfort or pain in the supporting hip, try bending the supporting knee more, increasing the pelvic tilt, or facing the support and using both hands to distribute the weight more evenly. If the pain persists try the seated alternative.

TECHNIQUE TIPS

Keep the supporting knee soft and over the ankle, the front leg and knee straight but not 'locked'.

✦

Keep the chest lifted as the leg lifts.

✦

Keep the breathing regular and natural. Perform slowly and with control.

SEATED ALTERNATIVE

✦ Sit tall with good posture. Your legs hip width apart, one knee bent over the ankle, the other leg straight out in front, heel on the floor, toe and knee facing the ceiling. Use a Dynaband (a special resistance band used for exercising) looped around the foot of the straight leg, held in the hands or secured against the chair seat. Straighten the knee against the resistance, hold for a second in the straight position. Bend and repeat as for the standing version opposite. (Bags of rice or traditional ankle weights can be used instead, to add resistance.) Always use the lightest Dynaband or weight to begin with and progress slowly.

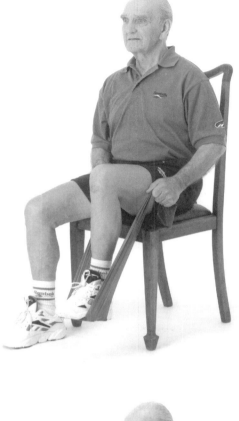

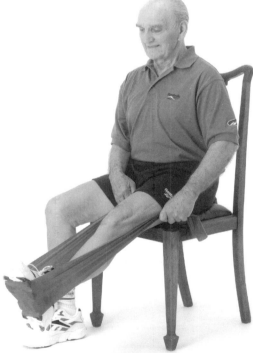

N.B. DAILY DOZEN no 11

Muscle Conditioning Plan

Lateral raise

PURPOSE

To condition the muscles at the top of the shoulders (deltoids) and
to strengthen the shoulder bones.

PREPARATION

✦ Stand or sit tall with good posture, with or without weights, your
knees bent, feet hip width apart and pointing forwards. Your
arms in front of your body, elbows slightly bent and palms facing
inwards. Increase your pelvic tilt, tighten tummy muscles.

ACTION

✦ Lift the arms outwards and upwards to the sides as far as possible
and then lower to the starting position. Keep the knees bent,
back long, tummy tight, elbows 'soft' and wrists straight.

Repeat until the arms tire. Rest with shoulder mobilisers (see page
71). As you get fitter, build up to a
maximum of 10 repetitions.

REPEAT X 2 MORE SETS.

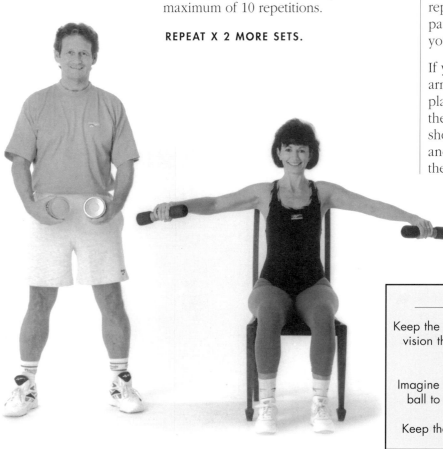

CAUTION

When using weights, never hold
your breath. Always move
slowly and with full control.
Avoid holding for long in any
position. Check posture
throughout.

If you have high blood pressure
check with your doctor before
using weights. Begin with light
weights, do a maximum of 6
repetitions and allow a generous
pause between each set until
your fitness improves.

If you have difficulty with any
arm moves above the shoulder,
place the arms and weights at
the sides of the thighs, lift the
shoulders up, hold for a second
and release with control back to
the start.

If you have arthritis in
the neck or shoulders
do not use weights for
this exercise.

TECHNIQUE TIPS

Keep the palms facing down and in your
vision throughout. Keep the shoulders
down and neck long.

✦

Imagine you are holding a giant beach
ball to get the soft curve in the arm.

✦

Keep the breathing regular and even.

The upward shoulder press

PURPOSE

To condition the muscles of the shoulders (deltoids and triceps) and strengthen the shoulder bones.

PREPARATION

✦ Stand or sit with good posture, with or without weights, legs hip width apart, knees bent and feet pointing forwards. Your arms bent up towards your shoulders, palms in a loose fist facing each other. If using weights, hold them securely. Increase your pelvic tilt and tighten your tummy muscles.

ACTION

✦ Press your arms straight up towards the ceiling, then lower to the starting position. Take care not to take the arms (and weights) out of your vision. Keep the elbows 'soft'. Avoid swinging into the move, use control from start to finish.

✦ Repeat for 6, or until the shoulders begin to tire. Rest and release tension by doing some shoulder circles (see page 71). As fitness grows, build to a maximum of 8 repetitions for strength, 15 for endurance.

REPEAT X 2 MORE SETS.

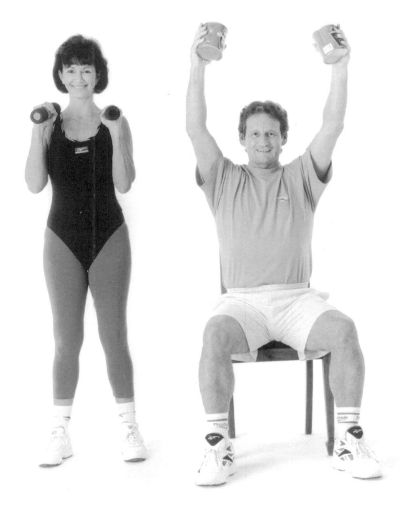

CAUTION

See Caution opposite.

TECHNIQUE TIPS

Keep the wrists straight and hold the weights firmly, but not tightly.

✦

Keep the breathing regular and even.

Back and spine strengtheners

PURPOSE

To condition the back muscles (erector spinae), improve posture and strengthen the spine.

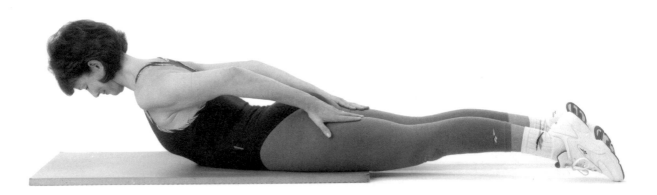

PREPARATION

✦ Lie face down on the floor with your legs together and your palms resting on your bottom. Do a pelvic tilt to lengthen your spine.

ACTION

✦ Keeping the spine and neck long, your forehead down and eyes looking at the floor, lift your shoulders off as far as you can. Hold briefly, return to the start. Lift and lower smoothly. Rest for a second.

✦ Repeat until your muscles begin to tire. Rest actively by doing the front-of-thigh stretch (page 122). As you get fitter, build up to a maximum of 10 repetitions in each set.

REPEAT X 3 MORE SETS.

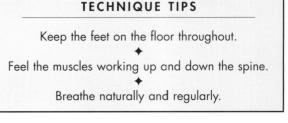

TECHNIQUE TIPS

Keep the feet on the floor throughout.
✦
Feel the muscles working up and down the spine.
✦
Breathe naturally and regularly.

CAUTION

If your lower back hurts during this exercise, place a folded towel under your hips to reduce the arch in your back. If it persists try the seated alternative.

If your hands feel uncomfortable try placing them on the floor beside your hips.

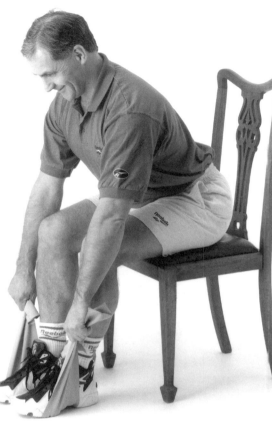

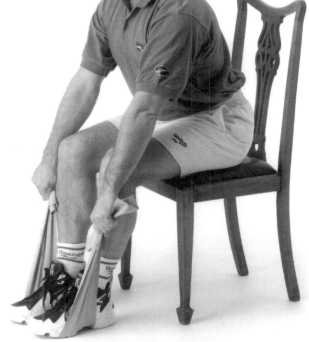

ALTERNATIVE

◆ Sit tall with good posture, legs and feet hip width apart, feet pointing forwards and slightly in front of the ankles, arms straight on either side of the legs, palms facing in with a weight in each hand, or a stretchy band under both feet with the ends held in each hand.

◆ Lean forward from the hips. Do a pelvic tilt, tighten the tummy muscles, lengthen your back upwards and lift against the resistance of the band. Do not allow your arms or shoulders to move backwards. This can be done without equipment. Hold for a count of 6. Lower with control.

REPEAT AND PROGRESS AS FOR THE LYING DOWN VERSION.

N.B. DAILY DOZEN no 12

Back leg lifts

PURPOSE

To condition the muscles at the back of the thigh (hamstrings) and bottom (gluteals), improve posture and strengthen the hip and thigh bones.

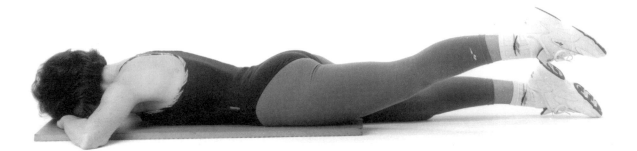

PREPARATION

✦ Lie on your front with your legs straight and together. Rest your forehead or chin on your hands for comfort. Increase the pelvic tilt and tighten the tummy muscles.

ACTION

✦ Lengthen one leg backwards along the floor, and tighten that buttock muscle. Keeping both hips pressed into the floor, and avoiding arching your back, lift the leg up a few inches, pause; lift again, pause and lower to the ground. Lower and lift with control. Keep the leg straight and think of lengthening and lifting rather than just lifting. Avoid leading with the heel – let the buttock muscles do the lifting.

✦ Repeat until your leg begins to tire. As fitness grows, build to a maximum of 12 repetitions. Repeat with other leg.

REPEAT X 2 MORE SETS.

TECHNIQUE TIPS

Avoid tensing the non-working leg.

✦

Feel the buttock and back of the thigh working.

✦

Keep the working hip pressed into the floor and your breathing even. Lower and lift with control.

CAUTION

If you feel discomfort in your back, try placing a folded towel under your hips. If it persists, avoid this exercise and try the seated alternative.

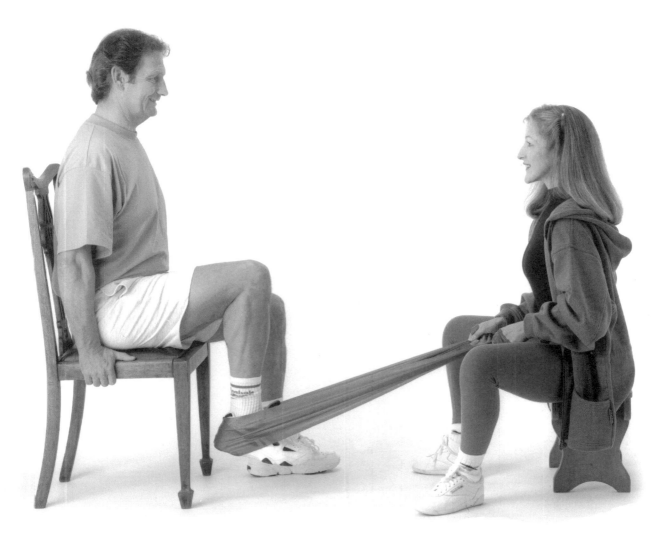

SEATED ALTERNATIVE

◆ Sit tall with good posture, your legs hip width apart and right foot slightly forward. Loop a dynaband around one heel. Tie ends to a heavy table leg, so they are secure – or get a friend to hold them. Holding your chair seat for support, tighten the abdominals and draw the heel backwards as far as you can against the resistance of the band. Feel the muscle work in the back of the thigh. Repeat as before.

Muscle Conditioning Plan

FLEXIBILITY STRETCHES PLUS

A unique feature of the Fitness For Life Plan is that there are flexibility stretches throughout the muscle conditioning to provide active 'rests' from the strength exercises and avoid any tension that may be felt when the stretches are done all together.

Lying front stretch

PURPOSE

To stretch the abdominal muscles (rectus abdominus) and mobilise the lower back.

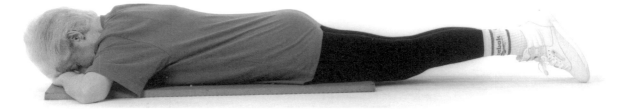

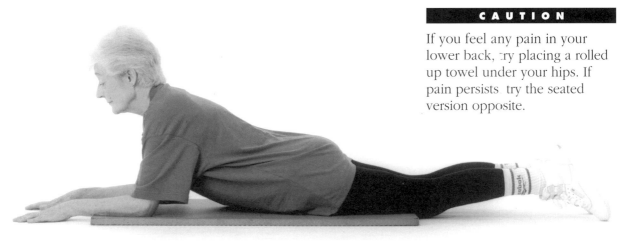

CAUTION

If you feel any pain in your lower back, try placing a rolled up towel under your hips. If pain persists try the seated version opposite.

PREPARATION

+ Lie on your front, your legs together, arms comfortably bent and forehead on your hands. Increase your pelvic tilt to prevent your back from arching.

+ Lift your upper body as you move your elbows into position directly under your shoulders; your forearms straight out in front, palms facing down, like a lion.

ACTION

+ Lengthen your body forwards and upwards by pressing down and pulling forwards against your shoulders and forearms, until you feel the stretch in the abdominals. Hold for a count of 10.

REST AND REPEAT X 1 MORE SET.

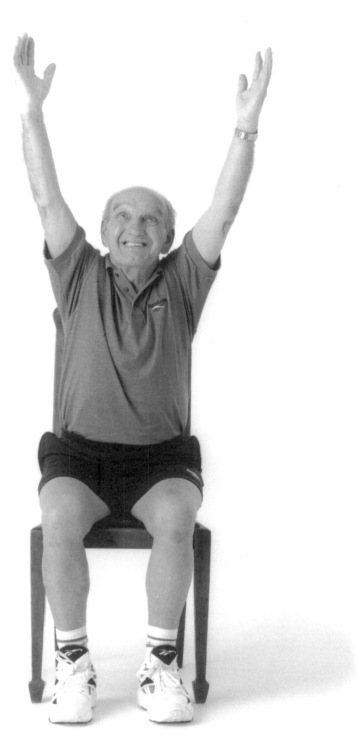

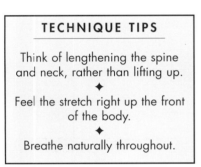

TECHNIQUE TIPS

Think of lengthening the spine and neck, rather than lifting up.

✦

Feel the stretch right up the front of the body.

✦

Breathe naturally throughout.

SEATED ALTERNATIVE

✦ Sit tall with good posture, your legs together, feet flat on the floor and palms on your thighs. Lean your upper body slightly forward from the hips. Pressing down through your feet, lengthen your upper body and spine upwards towards the ceiling, lifting the ribs as far away from the waist as you can. Hold as before.

Flying back lift

PURPOSE

To condition the muscles of the upper back and neck (trapezius and rhomboids), prevent rounded shoulders, and strengthen the upper spine.

> **TECHNIQUE TIPS**
>
> Take care not to hold the breath – very easy to do on this exercise.
>
> ✦
>
> Keep your legs on the floor throughout.
>
> ✦
>
> Feel that muscle work across the top of the back and shoulders.

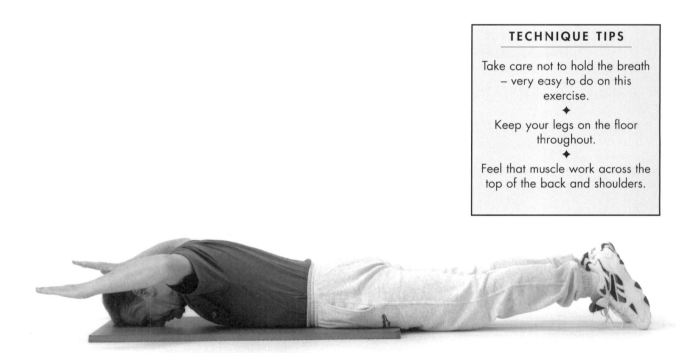

REPARATION

✦ Lie face down with your forehead on the mat, your legs hip width apart, and your arms straight out to the sides – just above shoulder height. Bend the forearms inwards, making a right angle at each elbow. Increase the pelvic tilt and tighten the tummy muscles.

ACTION

✦ Keeping your forehead on the mat and your neck long, lift your arms up, taking wrists and elbows towards the back of your head. Think of lengthening the spine as you lift the arms,

keeping the wrists in line with the elbows, and squeeze the shoulder blades together. Hold for a second and lower to the start.

✦ Repeat x 4 or until the muscles tire. Build to a maximum of 8.

REST AND REPEAT X 2 MORE SETS.

TO PROGRESS

Lying down: take the arms out to the sides just above shoulder height.

ALTERNATIVE

✦ Sit or stand tall with good posture, your legs hip width apart, knees bent and feet facing forward, your arms by your sides and weights held securely in your hands.

✦ Take your shoulders upwards, in a shrugging action. Hold for a second at the top of the movement, then take them downwards as far as possible. Hold for a second. Release and repeat, making the moves as large as possible.

Repeat as before.

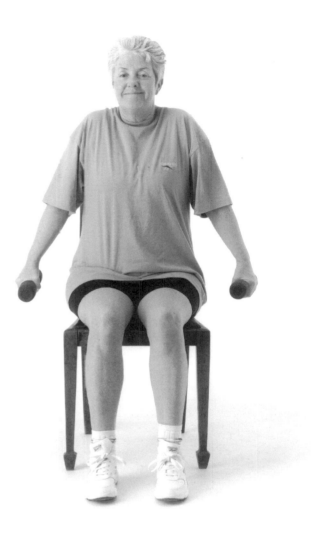

Front-of-thigh stretch

PURPOSE

To lengthen the muscles at the front of the thigh (quadriceps), to increase hip movement and counteract the shortening effects of sitting.

PREPARATION

✦ Lie face down, your legs straight and together, your forehead resting on your hands for comfort.

ACTION

✦ Lengthen the leg to be stretched, and bend the knee, bringing the heel towards your bottom. Take arm backwards on the same side of the body. Keeping a firm pelvic tilt to avoid arching your back, see if you can take hold of your ankle (or sock). If not, use a towel. You will feel a strong stretch down the front of your bent thigh. Re-tilt the pelvis if you need to increase the stretch.

✦ Hold for a count of 15-20. If the muscles give a little, and the stretching sensation fades, ease the leg in a little further to develop the stretch. Hold for a little longer. With control, release to the floor. Repeat with other leg.

REPEAT X 2 MORE SETS.

TECHNIQUE TIPS

Think of pressing the foot away from the bottom and retilting the pelvis. Avoid pulling the knee in towards the bottom.

✦

Ease particularly carefully and gradually into and out of this stretch. Breathe out as you ease into the stretch and keep your breathing natural throughout.

SEATED ALTERNATIVE

✦ Sit tall with good posture, sideways on the chair, both feet flat on the floor. Support yourself with one arm on the back of the chair. Keeping both hips facing forward, move your right leg carefully backwards along the front of the chair until your thigh and knee are behind the hip. Re-tilt your pelvis and feel the stretch as before. Hold for a count of 10. If comfortable, hold for longer as for lying version. Turn around and repeat on other side.

REPEAT X 2 MORE SETS.

CAUTION

Take particular care getting into and out of this longer stretch, using your free hand on the chair seat to assist in transferring your body weight.

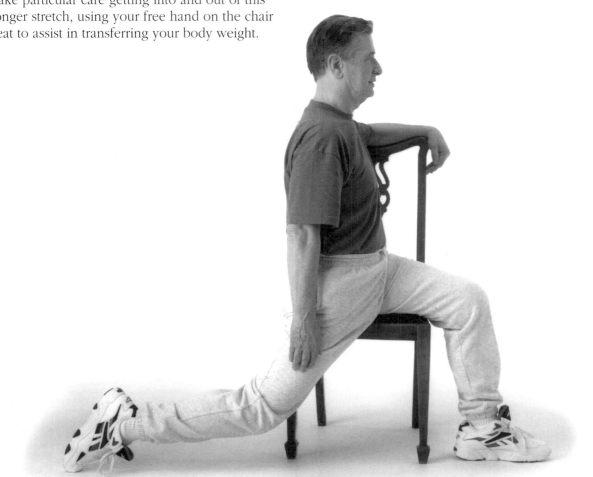

Outer thigh strengthener

PURPOSE

To condition the muscles on the outside of the hip and thigh (abductors), and strengthen the hip and thigh bones.

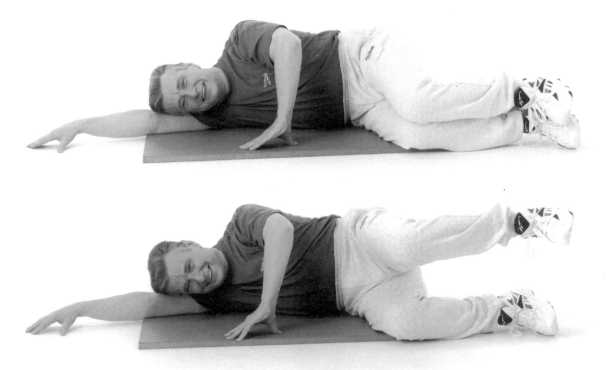

PREPARATION

✦ Lie on your left side. Bend both knees at a right angle to your hips, your ankles in line with the knees. Place your right hand on the floor in front of your chest for support, and rest your head on your left arm; alternatively, rest your head in your left hand. Check your posture and tighten your tummy muscles.

ACTION

✦ Keeping your hips facing forward, raise your right, bent leg, taking care not to let this hip roll backward. Hold for a second at the top of the movement, and lower to the start. Keep the knee and foot of the working leg facing the front, not the ceiling – otherwise you will be working the wrong muscles.

✦ Repeat until the muscles tire. Build up to a maximum of 12 repetitions. Rest by stretching left arm out in line with your head and doing a body stretch (page 129) on your side. Repeat with other thigh.

REPEAT X 2 MORE SETS.

TECHNIQUE TIPS

Try lengthening the top thigh towards the front before lifting.

✦

Feel the muscles working from the hip to the knee.

✦

Keep the breathing regular. Work with control.

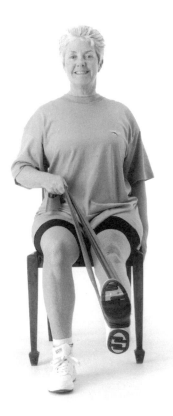
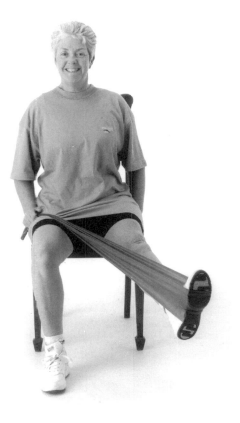

SEATED ALTERNATIVE

✦ Sit tall with good posture, legs hip width apart
and right leg straight out in front. Loop a
stretchy band once around the instep of that
foot. Keeping it taut, take the ends across the
thighs and hold them in the left hand, securing
them against the chair seat. Tightening the
tummy muscles and using the hands to support
the back, take the right leg out sideways away
from the body, pulling against the resistance of
the band. Return to start. Breathe evenly.
Repeat until the leg tires. Build to a maximum
of 6 repetitions. Rest by doing the abdominal
stretch on page 119. Repeat for other thigh.

REPEAT X 2 MORE SETS.

Basic lift ups

PURPOSE

To condition the abdominal muscles (rectus abdominis and obliques), to stabilise the back and assist the pelvic floor muscles.

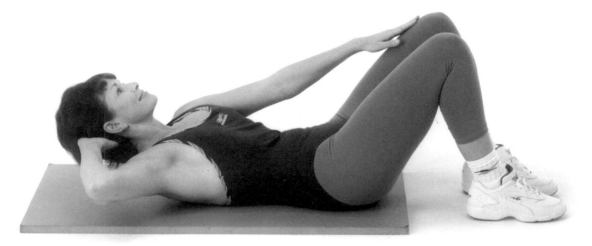

PREPARATION

✦ Lie on your back with your legs hip width apart, knees bent, feet flat on the floor, your head resting in your right hand and the left hand on your left thigh.

ACTION

✦ Do a firm pelvic tilt, breathe out and pull in your tummy muscles strongly throughout. Lift your shoulders off the floor and slide your fingertips along your thigh towards your knees. Make sure your neck is long, with a gap about the size of a grapefruit between your chin and your chest. Avoid pulling on the head, keep your shoulders down, elbows open and let the abdominals do the work. Ease back down to the start.

✦ Repeat slowly x 4. Rest by turning the head slowly side to side to release any tension in the neck. Build up to a maximum of 8 repetitions.

REPEAT X 2 MORE SETS.

TECHNIQUE TIPS

Take care in getting into position: use your arms to lower your body on to your side. Then use your feet on the floor to lower yourself on to your back.

✦

From time to time place your hand on your tummy; feel the muscles work in the abdomen.

✦

Breathe out as you tighten and lift up. **Breathe** in as you lower. Move slowly and with control.

CAUTION

If you feel any discomfort in your back, try placing a folded towel under the top of your thighs and bottom. If discomfort persists try the seated alternative.

If you have any rounding of the shoulders and your neck has to arch to allow your head to reach the floor, place a small cushion under your head.

CAUTION

If your neck hurts in the lying position you are tensing at the neck and leading with the chin, instead of letting the abdominals do the work. Try consciously softening the neck muscles and/or put both hands behind the head. Alternatively, go back to the Basic Pelvic Tilt (see page 57) and pull in until your muscles are stronger.

Never lift too high – only the shoulder blades should lift off the floor.

Never perform sit ups with your legs straight.

SEATED ALTERNATIVE

✦ Sit tall, your legs and feet hip width apart and your knees bent. Increase the pelvic tilt and breathe out as you pull the tummy muscles in strongly towards your spine. Keep the chest lifted and shoulders relaxed. Hold for a count of 6. If you run out of breath before you get to 6 then just breathe normally. Relax for a moment and start the exercise again. Repeat and rest as for lying version.

REPEAT X 2 SETS.

✦ For ease and variety, lie on your back and rest your lower legs on the seat of a chair.

Lying back-of-thigh stretch

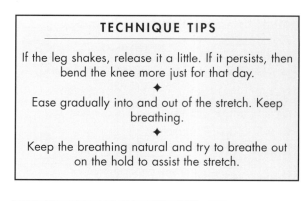

PURPOSE

To lengthen the muscles at the back of the thigh (hamstrings). To prevent stiffness in the hip, legs, spine and lower back.

PREPARATION

✦ Lie on your back with both knees bent and both feet flat on the floor.

ACTION

✦ Bend the knee of the leg to be stretched in towards your chest; place one hand on the back of the thigh and the other on the calf. Allow the muscles to release a little.

✦ Straighten the leg upwards as you press gently with the hands on the leg, easing it in towards you until you feel a stretch in the back of the thigh. Take care not to pull, force or bounce the stretch. Avoid lifting the base of your spine and buttocks off the floor. Keep both hips facing the ceiling and the leg in line with the hip to avoid twisting the back. Keep the head and shoulders on the floor, the spine and neck long and relaxed.

✦ Hold for a count of 30. If the muscles give a little and the stretch becomes easier, ease the leg in a little further and hold for a little longer. If not, then come out of the stretch, rest and repeat. Repeat for the other leg. Avoid clasping the hands together behind the thigh.

REPEAT TWICE MORE

TECHNIQUE TIPS

If the leg shakes, release it a little. If it persists, then bend the knee more just for that day.

✦

Ease gradually into and out of the stretch. Keep breathing.

✦

Keep the breathing natural and try to breathe out on the hold to assist the stretch.

CAUTION

If you are fairly tight in the hamstrings so that it is difficult to keep your leg into your chest, loop a towel round your ankle to support the leg. Ease it in as before. If you still feel any discomfort in your lower back, try the seated alternative.

If you have an artificial hip, use the towel and do not bring the leg past a 90° angle at the hip.

SEATED ALTERNATIVE

See Back-of-Thigh Stretch on page 134.

Full body stretch

PURPOSE

To elongate the muscles in a supported position.

PREPARATION

✦ Lie on your back with knees bent and feet flat on the floor, arms at your sides. Do a pelvic tilt to lengthen your back along the floor and tighten the tummy muscles.

✦ Keeping your back on the floor slide your right foot along the floor to straighten the leg. Straighten the left leg in the same way.

✦ Take your arms over your head and rest them on the floor.

ACTION

✦ Stretch the whole length of your body, taking the fingertips and toes as far away from the centre as possible. Avoid taking the chin to the ceiling or arching the back; keep the spine and neck long. Feel the stretch all along the front and sides of your body.

✦ Hold for a second then completely let go – releasing and softening the muscles. Repeat as often as you like.

SEATED ALTERNATIVE

✦ Sit tall, your legs together, knees bent, feet flat on the floor, your arms over your head, palms facing inward. Keeping the lower body still, your neck and back long, reach for the sky elongating ribs, arms and fingertips upwards. Then take a firm hold of your chair seat and with your toes resting on the floor, lengthen your legs out along the ground. Release and rest for 30 seconds.

REPEAT ONCE MORE.

If you have difficulty taking your arms over your head, take them out to the sides as high or low as is comfortable.

If doing the seated alternative, leave your arms in the air for a count of about 3 and then release.

The diagonal lift up

PURPOSE

To condition the abdominal muscles (obliques, rectus abdominis), stabilise the back and assist the pelvic floor muscles.

PREPARATION

✦ Lie on your back with your legs hip width apart, knees bent and feet flat on the floor; your head resting in your left hand and your right hand palm down on the floor, at about chest height. Do a firm pelvic tilt.

ACTION

✦ Keeping the left elbow back behind the ear, pull in your tummy muscles strongly and lift your shoulder, twisting slightly towards your right knee. Ease back down to the start. Keep the shoulders down, chest open and lifted away from the waist, both hips on the floor.

✦ Repeat x 4 or until the muscles tire. Build up to a maximum of 8. Then repeat on the other side. Rest by circling the wrists.

REPEAT X 2 SETS.

Technique Tips and Cautions as for the BASIC LIFT UPS (pages 126–127).

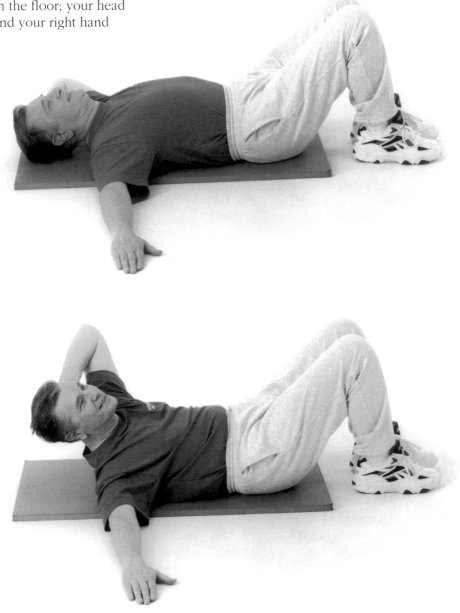

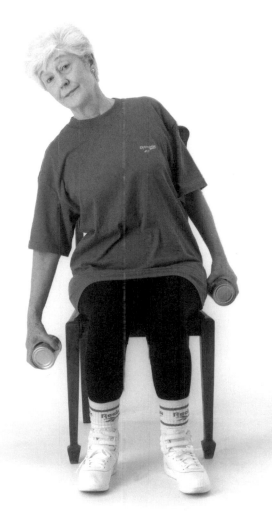

TECHNIQUE TIPS

Feel the muscles on the straight
side working hard to lift you
back to the centre.

◆

Breathe out as you lower the
body to the side and lift
back to centre.

ALTERNATIVE

◆ Sit or stand tall, your legs and feet hip width apart, knees bent.
Hold a weight securely in both hands, arms at the side of your
thighs. Do a pelvic tilt, pull in your tummy muscles strongly
throughout and keep your shoulders down as you lift the upper
body up, and over to one side. Keep the arm in line with the hip
and avoid leaning forwards or backwards. Return to the centre.
Repeat to other side. Follow repetitions suggested opposite.

Back-of-thigh stretch

PURPOSE

To lengthen the muscles at the back of the thigh (hamstrings).

PREPARATION

✦ Sit tall with good posture, near the edge of your chair, legs hip width apart and knees bent over the ankles.

ACTION

✦ Straighten one leg out in front of you, resting your heel on the floor. Place both hands just above the bent knee to support your back and body weight. Lift the chest and lengthen the whole upper body upwards and forwards until you feel a stretch in the back of the straight thigh.

✦ Hold for a count of 10; release and repeat on the other side.

REPEAT ONCE MORE.

TECHNIQUE TIPS

If you can't feel the stretch, try tilting your bottom upwards a little but avoid arching your back.

✦

If you feel the stretch in the calf, take your toes nearer to the floor.

✦

Ease gradually into and out of the stretch. Keep breathing even.

CAUTION

If you find your back is rounded and you are unable to sit tall, place a folded towel under your bottom.

RELAX for a moment or two using the relaxation techniques in Chapter 4. This furthers the **cool-down** process, adds to the benefit of the workout and enhances the final seated stretches.

Inner thigh stretch

PURPOSE

To lengthen the muscles of the inner thigh (adductors) and improve hip movement.

PREPARATION

Sit tall on the floor or chair, soles of feet together, your back long and chest lifted (or ankles crossed or even legs shoulder-width apart or wider, knees bent and feet flat on the floor), arms placed comfortably along the inside thighs. Allow your knees to flop apart.

ACTION

✦ Use your arms and hands to press your thighs open and down until you feel a stretch along the inner thigh.

✦ Hold for a count of 30. If the muscles give a little, ease a little further into the stretch and hold for a little longer. If not, come out of the stretch. Rest.

REPEAT TWICE MORE.

TECHNIQUE TIPS

Ease gradually into and out of the stretch. Breathe naturally throughout and try to breathe out on the hold to assist the stretch.

✦

Comfort is really important so try the alternatives to find what suits you.

✦

In the floor version, hold your *ankles*, not your toes.

Trunk and chest stretch

PURPOSE

To stretch the abdominal muscles (obliques), to improve range of movement in the neck, shoulders and spine.

PREPARATION

✦ Sit tall with good posture, legs hip width apart, knees bent over your ankles, and your feet facing forward.

ACTION

✦ Place your right hand on your left knee and lengthen your body upwards. Turn your upper body towards your left arm and place this arm on the back of the chair.

✦ Lengthen your spine upwards again and turn your body a little further to the back. Use the hand on your knee to help ease yourself into position. Take care to keep the hips facing forward and the thighs and knees hip width apart. Avoid forcing the stretch by pushing on the knee or chair back. Keep the shoulders down and chest open. Feel the stretch across the front and sides of the upper body.

✦ Hold for a count of 10. Release and return to centre. Do a pelvic roll to refresh the back and repeat on the other side.

REPEAT ONCE MORE.

Complete your muscle conditioning workout by repeating the Back of Arm Stretch (page 91) and the Upward Side Stretch (page 88).

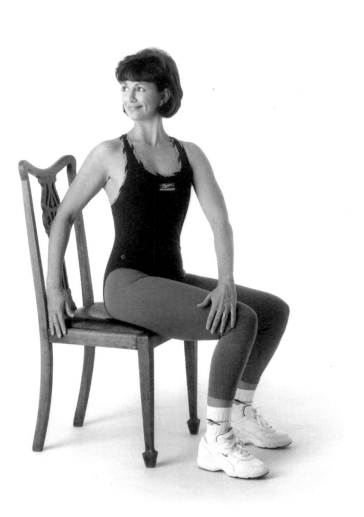

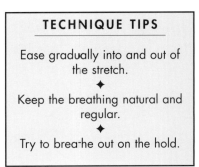

TECHNIQUE TIPS

Ease gradually into and out of the stretch.

✦

Keep the breathing natural and regular.

✦

Try to breathe out on the hold.

Relaxation

If you have the opportunity for a fuller relaxation –
treat yourself! Get really comfortable and follow the
techniques in Chapter 4.

Remobilisers

To ensure you finish alert and focused,
'remobilise' with some shoulder lifts and
circles. First perform these seated to allow
your circulation to adjust and then, in your
own time and way, get carefully to your feet
and repeat them again. Finish with some Easy
Walks (page 69) then a final whole body
stretch (the Free Style Reach below).

Free style reach

ACTION

◆ Lengthen your arms and body upwards or outwards at
shoulder level as if doing a giant yawn – or whatever
movement pleases you. A chance to move freely and do
your own thing! Repeat 3 times, then take a long breath in
and out. You should feel relaxed and refreshed.

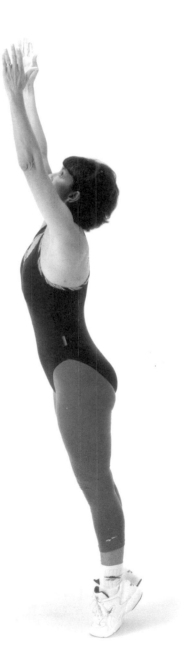

CHAPTER

7

The art of active living

You will soon be delighted by the difference regular exercise makes to your life. By also consciously applying the posture tips, exercise and relaxation techniques to everyday situations you will benefit much more than if you think about them only once or twice a week.

Every time we are lazy about such actions as straightening up to our full height when getting out of a chair, we lose vital strength and length in our muscles. Every time we pick up a heavy object without bending our knees, we risk straining muscles and ligaments, and jarring joints. Gradually we lose the fine tuning of skill, co-ordination and balance required to complete the action with control. What a waste, when each daily move is an opportunity to work on our posture, conserve energy, lessen joint wear and tear, and to take a pride in our increased body awareness and agility.

Once we practise the correct way to do these everyday transitions, it is amazing how economical and natural they feel – and how much stronger our muscles become. The trick is to catch ourselves just as we are about to throw our bodies into something. Stop and think – 'there must be a better way'.

Getting from A to B less disgracefully

Standing to sitting (on the floor)
Stand tall with good posture behind, and to one side of, a chair, with your legs and feet hip width apart, the nearer hand on the back of the chair and the other by your side. Take a small stride forward alongside the chair, with the leg which is nearer the support; your back heel will be lifted. Distribute your weight evenly between your legs and, using

the chair-back for balance and support, lower your back knee to the ground. Release your back toe, so the foot is flat to prevent cramp. Thinking tall, take the other knee to the floor. Move the chair to the front of your body and place one arm on the chair seat and the other on the floor to lower your weight until you are sitting legs to one side on the floor. Tighten the tummy muscles and take the legs round, one at a time, until you are sitting, legs hip width apart and knees bent. Practise until you can do this beside the chair but almost without using it.

Then progress to free standing. Take the stride forward as before and place both hands on the front knee to support your weight as you lower yourself, thinking tall, to the floor. Take your arms to your sides, get your balance and then take the knee to the floor. Then lower your bottom to one side and finally bring your legs round.

Sitting to lying (on the floor)

Sit tall on the floor and bend your knees up comfortably with your feet flat on the floor. Turn your body towards your stronger side and use your arms to lower yourself down to lie on that side. Pull your knees in further and keeping your feet in contact with the floor, roll smoothly on to your back and walk your feet round until they are hip width apart, your back long and your shoulders, hips and feet in line.

Lying to sitting

Simply reverse the above. With your knees bent and feet flat on the floor, roll over to lie on your stronger side, bring the knees in further and still lying side on, push up from the floor with your arms. Take your top arm over and place it on the floor beside your hip to support your back as you bring your body to face forward.

Lying with bent knees to lying with straight legs

Do a pelvic tilt to lengthen your back along the floor, tighten your tummy muscles and slide one foot along the floor until the leg is straight. Check the tilt and repeat with the other leg. Lift the head and check your 'plumb line' (a straight line that should run from your head and chin to your pubic bone).

Sitting (on the floor) to standing

Sitting tall, knees bent and the chair on your strong arm side, use your arms to support you as you place one arm on the chair seat and the other on the floor by your hip. Take your knees towards the chair. Then, taking the hand near the hip and placing it on the floor in front of your knees, use both arms to support you to kneeling. Take one knee forward, placing your foot flat on the floor. Do a pelvic tilt, tighten your tummy, count to three, and in one move press down with the thigh muscles of the bent knee. Bring the other leg alongside and, steadying yourself against the chair seat, stand halfway up. Then straighten both knees and come up completely. Practise this as before.

Then progress to free standing. Place the knees and feet to one side as before, using one hand on the floor to push up to a kneeling position. Take one knee up and place one foot flat on the floor. Steadying yourself with both hands on one knee, tighten the tummy, think tall, count three and press down with both thighs to stand. Bring both legs together, knees bent, and then lengthen to stand tall.

Once you have mastered this on your strong side, begin on your weaker side.

Sitting (on a chair) to standing

Sit tall at the front of the chair, your legs hip width apart and your feet facing forwards slightly further back than usual, your toes directly under your knees and heels on the floor, your hands resting lightly on your thighs. Lean forward and upwards, beginning to take your weight more over your thighs, do a pelvic tilt and tighten your tummy muscles. Prepare to stand after a count of three. Keeping your head up press down strongly and swiftly through your thighs and feet, push lightly on your hands and stand straight up. Think up, not forwards, and let your thighs do all the work. Build this to a rhythm and finally do it without the hands. Then take the feet further forward as this is harder. (See page 107.)

Standing to sitting (on a chair)

Stand tall, with your palms resting on your thighs. Do a pelvic tilt and tighten the tummy muscles and, keeping the knees over the toes, stick your bottom out slightly and, keeping your hands on your thighs, lower yourself to the chair. Think of lengthening upwards even though you are travelling backwards. Move with control, especially the last inch – don't give in and let go.

Lifting technique

One of the main sources of back injuries arises from incorrect lifting technique and poor abdominal control. The main function of the abdominals is to act as a splint for the lumbar spine. Weak abdominals and tight back muscles leave the lower back vulnerable.

The main problem however, is the angle of the body in relation to the object being lifted. Instead of bending the knees and taking the strain through the strong, large thigh muscles, most people tend to bend forward from the hips and keep their legs straight as they reach over to pick up the object. This is usually one unthinking move, often with the arms fully or partially extended as they lift. The added strain of the forward flexed trunk, the lengthened lever of the arms, multiplies the weight being lifted many times, and places immense strain on the delicate ligaments and muscles of the lower back. The further away the arms from the trunk, the more dangerous the move is for the back. Adding a twist to the movement is a recipe for injury and possibly months of pain. Good lifting technique, and strong abdominals, can prevent these unnecessary injuries.

The lifting phase/the pick up

Stand as near to the object as possible with your hips square and feet pointing slightly outwards. Bend your knees, keeping them in line with the toes, the back long and head erect. Draw the object in towards the centre of your body. Tighten the abdominals, count to three and push up strongly through the thighs, still holding the object close.

Lowering phase

Reverse the lifting action. Having reached your destination, steady yourself, tighten the abdominals and, keeping the back long, bend the knees to lower the object to the floor. Release the object, place your hands on your thighs, count three and stand up, pushing up through the thighs as before.

Use this technique for all lifting and lowering actions, no matter how light the object.

Telephone tips

We should feel comfortable when using the telephone. A warm, draught-free spot, a high-backed chair with long arm rests to support the head, neck and arms; sitting well back in the chair with both feet on the ground; changing the receiver side occasionally and keeping the breathing regular, all help to reduce postural stress. Taking one easy breath in and out before we speak at the start of the conversation, and softening our shoulders, helps us to **respond** instead of react, especially if the conversation is a difficult one.

Driving tips

Tiredness and tension cause accidents. We need to be alert yet relaxed. Checking our seat height and distance from the pedals, sitting well back in the seat, using cushions to add extra support if necessary, are important. The muscles and spine respond best to change; varying the cushion positions occasionally, moving gently and constantly and, on long journeys getting out and walking briskly for four to five minutes every hour or so, revitalises the brain and body.

Changing your hand grip as you turn the steering wheel allows your spine to be as straight as possible against the support. If your elbows are loose at your sides and your hands maintain a comfortably firm hold, rather than grasping the wheel tightly, your whole posture will be one of easy, supported length, so you can steer smoothly and respond readily with a minimum of tension. If you are held up, never fret or do battle with other drivers but breathe deeply, turn your head from side to side and open your mouth, 'freeing' the jaw to release tension.

Getting in and out of cars can be an exercise in efficiency and elegant economy of movement, or ungainly, all-revealing and even dangerous. Remember to sit tall with tight abdominals and a long spine; use your arms to help swing both legs to the side of the car. Changing the hand, hold to either side of your body, count to three, and push up strongly through your thighs to standing. Reverse this process to get into the car.

Gardening tips

Back care is a major concern when gardening. Always use correct lifting technique and never sit back on your heels, particularly not on wet grass. Using a low stool and long handled tools can prevent back and knee strain. Getting up, stretching and walking about at regular intervals, prevents stiffness and circulation problems. Vary the activity after 30 minutes if it is unfamiliar; do a little of several jobs on one evening. In this way, by the end of the week all the jobs will be done without excessive strain on weak muscles. And always take a few minutes rest every 30 minutes or so.

Bath tips

Getting in and out of the bath can be hazardous, if you do so without due care. Begin by sitting on a small towel on the edge of the bath. Then, keeping both knees together, swivel both legs round towards one end until the nearer leg is touching the bath. Using the outside leg for support, tightening the tummy muscles and lengthening upwards, lift the other leg into the bath. Lift the remaining leg across to sit on the bath side with the feet in the water. Lean across the bath and place one hand firmly on the opposite side and turn the body slightly towards the top end again. Take a firm hold of the bath side with both hands and, again tightening the tummy muscles, count three and lower the body into the water. Reverse these actions to get out. If standing up is difficult, the safest way to get out is to get on to the hands and knees and hold on to the side for support. A rubber mat on the bottom of the bath is a must.

Night time tips

Whether we are wakeful at the beginning or middle of the night, we usually discover muscle tension throughout our bodies, and a more rapid breathing pattern. Suddenly, the fear tension reflex is triggered, worries flood in and we are wide awake.

A combination of getting up, walking briskly around the house for five minutes, stretching and settling a little before using relaxation techniques, all help to quieten our muscles and ease tension. Daytime catnapping is an invaluable way to restore energy or prepare for a special night out!

Active living – the workout of life

The Fitness For Life approach offers something for everyone and every occasion. We leave you to examine your life for opportunities to use the exercise techniques and training tips. As you have seen, even when exercise has no appeal, or on those days when you cannot manage a workout – everyday living can keep you on the move and be a workout in itself. Just doing the vacuuming or washing the car, for example, we could go at it with more gusto than usual and try to make it continuous; briskly make the backwards and forwards sweeps and change arms occasionally to balance the muscle conditioning. Even brushing our teeth in the morning can turn into a vigorous experience as we make bigger strokes, change hands, and

add a Balance or an Easy Walk! When we have to go upstairs for something, we could add to that daily 30 minute activity quota by doing it four times. The possibilities are endless and this active living approach can really make a difference to your health.

Active living and lifestyle

Fitness gives us the opportunity of a full life, a Body Age that is years younger than our actual age, a health span and physical capacity that extends to match our Life Span, and a confidence, energy and enjoyment of life that is ageless. Without doubt fitness is at its most effective in achieving physical health when it is combined with healthy eating and other lifestyle changes, such as giving up smoking, drinking in moderation and reducing the frenetic pace of our lives. The great thing about regular exercise and an active lifestyle is that, without thinking about it, you start to move nearer to looking at, reviewing and finally, ringing the changes in these other lifestyle factors. All in good time and one thing at a time. The important thing is to begin to put the activity back into your life today.

Our activity choices must be right for us, our bodies and our lives. For some of us, taking exercise may be a way to get some fresh air, enjoy nature and find solitude. For others it may be a chance to discover the gym and the company of like-minded people. It may be that at different times we will want all these things. We need to vary our programme, review it against our goals, be gentle with ourselves and above all enjoy it. Remember it doesn't matter how little you do at first, as even the smallest bit counts towards that Activity Total. The one golden rule is that you do it, and start today! 'Use it or lose it' – it's a powerful choice!

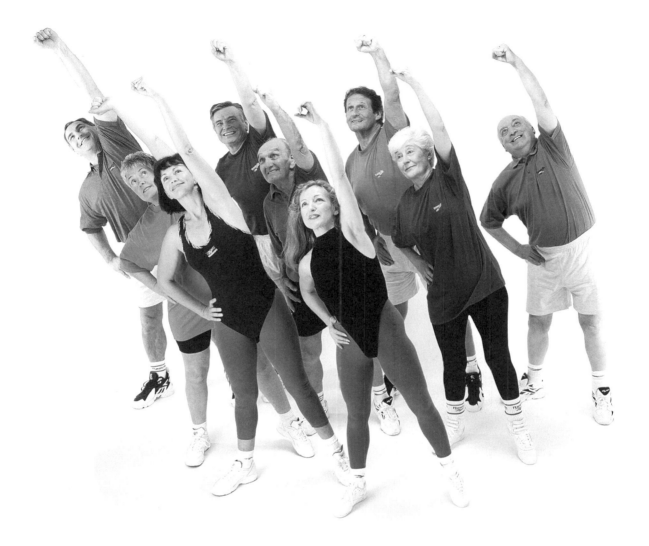

Age-ility!

With thanks to our real-life models (from the back row, left to right):
Bob Hope (46), Bill Elliot (68), Peter Thomas (53), George Banks (75), Dolly Taylorson (54),
Ben Ely (84), Diana Barnes (72), Babs Thomas (46) and Susie Dinan (47).

Resources

Recommended Further Reading

Energise For Exercise Penny Hunking, (published by Penny Hunking). Available from Energise, PO Box 244, Woking, Surrey, GU22 7FD.

Aquarobics Glenda Baum (Arrow Books)

Fitness Walking Therese Iknoian (Human Kinetics)

Fitness Weight Training Thomas Baechle & Roger Earle (Human Kinetics)

Recommended Videos

Easy Does It (Lifetime Productions). Part of the *Fitness Club* range of exercise videos available from Central YMCA Training & Development Dept, 112 Great Russell Street, London WC1B 3NQ. Telephone 0171 580 2989.

The Easy Going Workout (BMG Video). Part of the *Fitness Club* range of exercise videos by Central YMCA (see above).

The Y Plan Countdown (VVL Video). Part of the *Y Plan* series of exercise videos by Central YMCA (see above).

Prime Time (Blackbird Productions). Available from The Exercise Association of England (see below).

Qualified Teachers

To find a qualified fitness teacher contact the Exercise Association of England (EXA) Unit 4, Angel Gate, 326 City Road, London EC1V 2PT. Telephone 0171 278 0811.

If you would like to become a qualified fitness teacher, contact Central YMCA (see above).

Equipment

For Dynabands, weights etc, contact Pro Active Health, Oxford Airport, Longford Lane, Kidlington, Oxon OX5 1RA. Telephone 01865 370778.

Useful Addresses

Central YMCA, Training and Development Department, 112 Great Russell Street, London WC1B 3NQ. Telephone 0171 580 2989

Age Concern England, Astral House, 1268 London Road, Newbury, London SW16 4ER. Telephone 0181 679 8000.

Ramblers Association, 1/5 Wandsworth Road, London SW8 2XX.

Index